Learn about

5 Steps Towards managing Aches and Pains

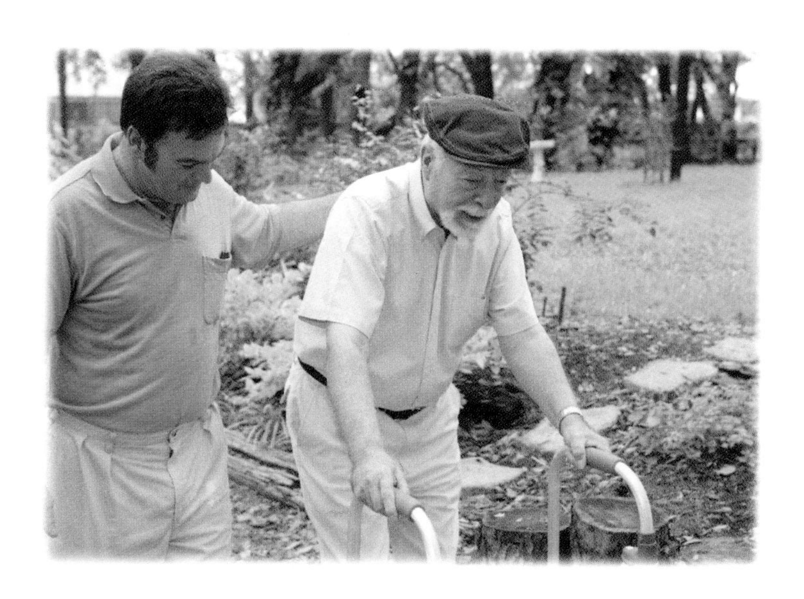

Learn about

5 Steps Towards managing Aches and Pains

Dr. ANJALI ARORA

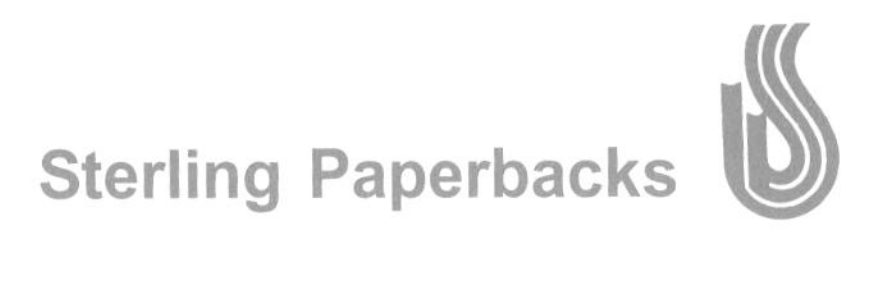

STERLING PAPERBACKS
An imprint of
Sterling Publishers (P) Ltd.
A-59, Okhla Industrial Area, Phase-II,
New Delhi-110020.
Tel: 26387070, 26386209; Fax: 91-11-26383788
E-mail: mail@sterlingpublishers.com
www.sterlingpublishers.com

5 Steps Towards
Managing Aches and Pains

arora_doc@hotmail.com
ISBN 978 81 207 4919 1

The author wishes to thank all academicians, scientists and writers who have been a source of inspiration.

The author and publisher specifically disclaim any liability, loss or risk, whatsoever, personal or otherwise, which is incurred as a consequence, directly or indirectly of the use and application of any of the contents of this book.

Printed and Published by Sterling Publishers Pvt. Ltd.,
New Delhi-110020.

Contents

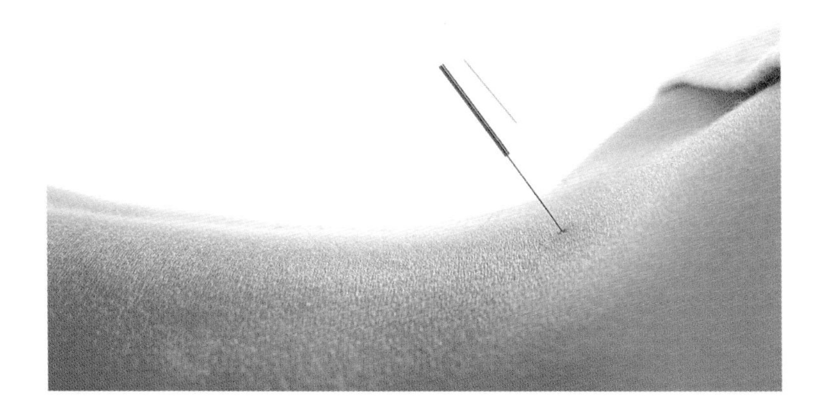

Find Out the Level of Your Awareness About Aches and Pains

1. **Pain in knees can be partially relieved by**
   a. Putting on weight
   b. Losing weight
   c. Just sitting the whole day
2. **Sleeping on a foam mattress for long duration**
   a. Is good for the back
   b. Is bad for the back
   c. Does not make a difference
3. **Muscle aches and pains can be due to the intake of medication like**
   a. Analgesics
   b. Statins
   c. Zyloric
4. **Leg cramps normally occur due to**
   a. Headache
   b. Electrolyte imbalance
   c. An injury

The above questionnaire will help you find out as to how aware you are about your aches and pains. If you answer more of (b) then you know how to help yourself.

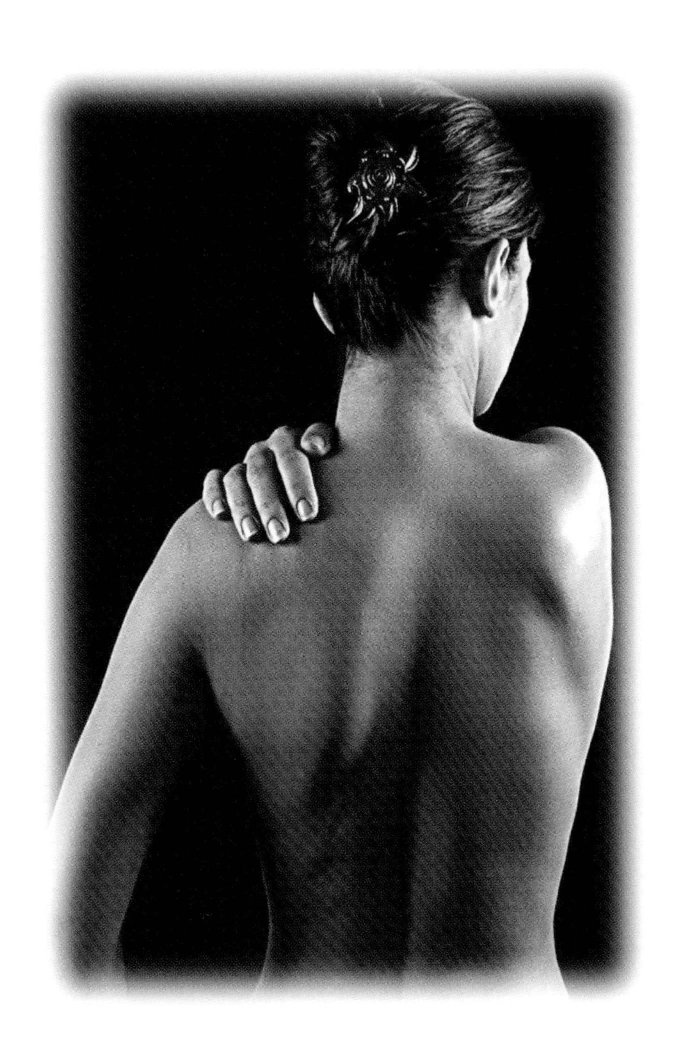

1 Arthritis and The Joints

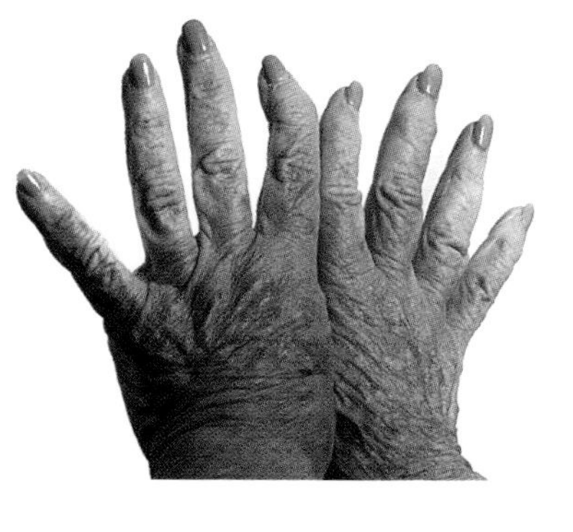

The body's 206 bones are connected through different types of joints. These different kinds of joints perform various functions. Some of these joints are:

- The ball and socket joints (hips and shoulders)
- Hinge joints (e.g. help connecting knees)
- Pivot joints (wrist)
- Saddle joints (connecting the thumb to the hand)
- Vertebral joints

The joints are tied together by ligaments and covered with cartilage. The cartilage is smooth, but made up of tough, elastic material. It acts as a shock absorber and allows the bone ends to glide smoothly across each other. A joint cavity exists between the bones. This gives the bone the room to move. The joint space between the bones is enclosed by a capsule. The inner lining of this capsule,

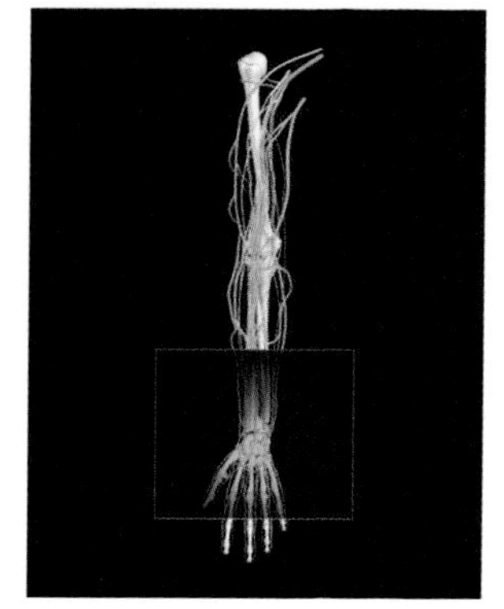

is the synovium, which produces a thick fluid that helps lubricate and nourish the joints.

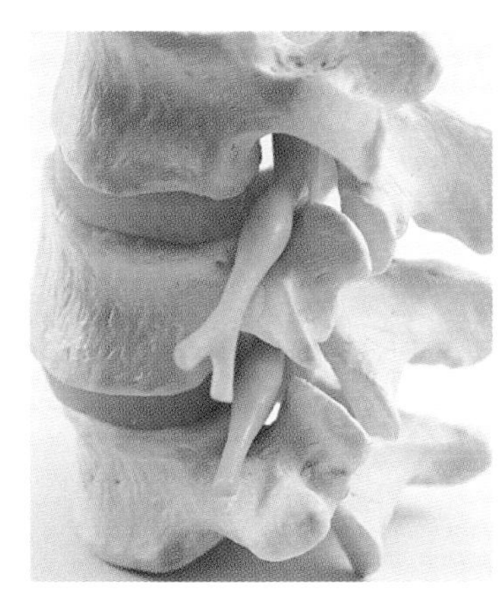

Arthritis

Primary Forms of Arthritis

- Osteoarthritis
- Rheumatoid arthritis
- Gout and pseudogout
- Septic arthritis
- Juvenile idiopathic arthritis
- Ankylosing spondylitis
- Still's disease

Secondary Forms of Arthritis

- Psoriatic arthritis
- Lupus erythematosus
- Reactive arthritis

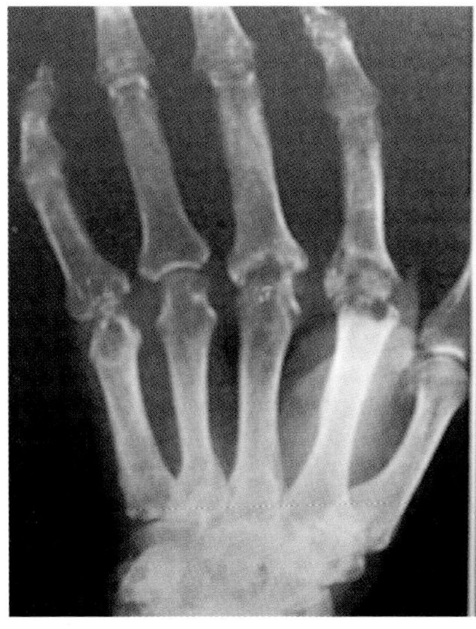

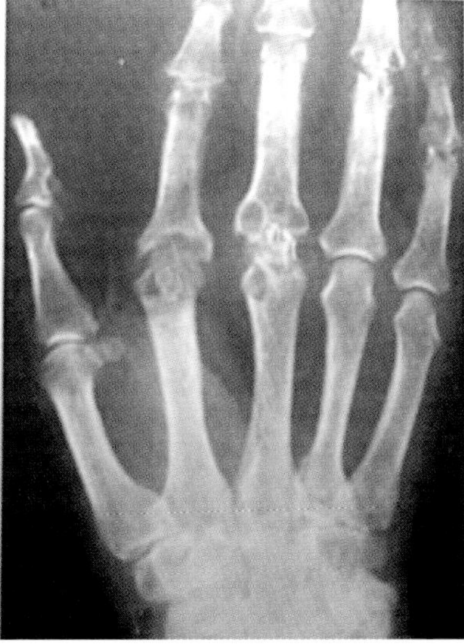

Some diseases which present themselves like arthritis are : -

- Osteoporosis
- Multiple myeloma
- Hypertrophic osteoarthropathy

Osteoarthritis

Osteoarthritis is basically an ailment of the joints. Osteoarthritis is not a primary inflammatory disorder, but is due to the gradual wear and tear of the affected area. Pathologically, osteoarthritis is defined as loss of articular cartilage and damage of the bone.

Osteoarthritis (OA) can be Primary or Secondary

Primary OA – The cause of osteoarthritis is primarily related to ageing. Primary osteoarthritis occurs without any identifiable cause.

Secondary OA – It is normally due to the presence of an underlying condition or disease like

- Injury to joint from an accident
- Inflammatory disorder, e.g. septic arthritis

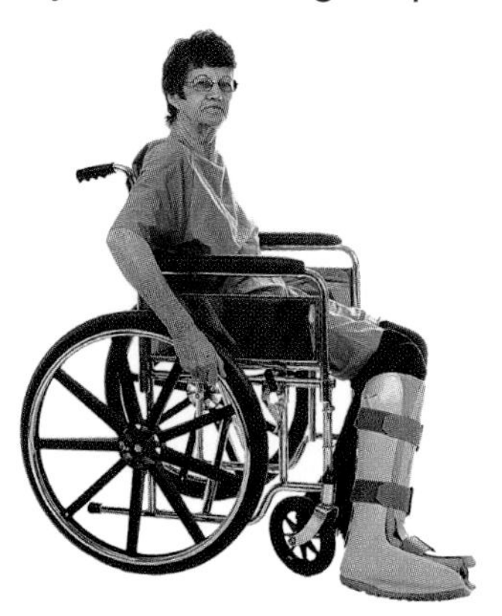

- Deficiency disorder as bow leg
- Metabolic condition, e.g. acromegaly

Symptoms of Osteoarthritis

Osteoarthritis symptoms start appearing in middle age. Around 65 years of age most people get affected by it. It is more common in women around 55 years of age.

- OA which presents itself with pain and stiffness in the joints is due to the presence of a low grade inflammation.
- The wear and tear of the cartilage (which normally acts as cushion) inside the joint results in this disease. The decrease of synovial fluid lubricating the joint also gets affected.
- Weight bearing like standing and walking causes pain in the joints. Less protection of the bones by the cartilage, results in this malady.
- Pain reduces movement of the joint resulting in atrophy of muscles around the joint. The ligaments in the affected area also become less elastic.
- New pieces of bones can grow around the margins of the joints (spurs or osteophytes). These bony changes along with the inflammation can lead to a painful and debilitating osteoarthritic condition.

Diagnosis of osteoarthritis is normally through X-rays and MRI. The incidence of osteoarthritis increases with age.

Treatment of Osteoarthritis

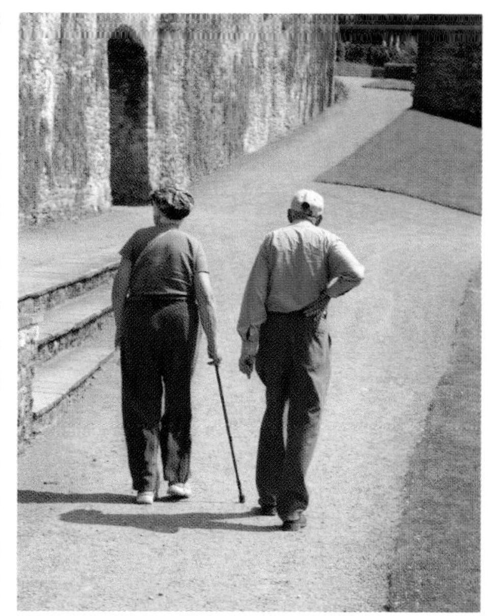

Rubefacients, emollients or topical analgesics are used in sprains, strains, lower back pain, and rheumatic pain. The ingredients include salicylates, nicotinates, histamine, etc. Their application often causes a local sensation of warmth. Menthol and camphor in the rubefacient produces coolness.

Medication

- NSAIDS (non-steroidal anti-inflammatory drugs)
- Local injections of glucocorticoids
- Omega 3 fatty acids
- Antioxidants (Vitamin C and E)
- Other specific medication as required.

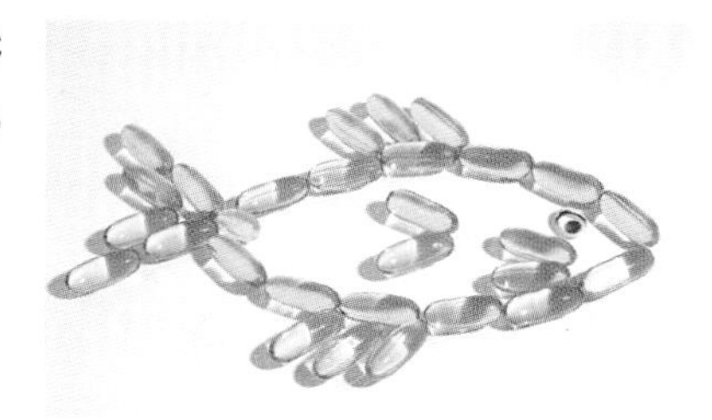

Supportive Treatment

- Weight loss
- A walker can be helpful
- Regular exercise (walking, swimming)
- Moist heat helps easing pain and swelling and can improve circulation.

Other Forms of Treatment Include:

- Acupuncture
- Low level laser therapy
- Radiosynovirothesis (a radioactive isotope is introduced into the joint to soften the tissue).

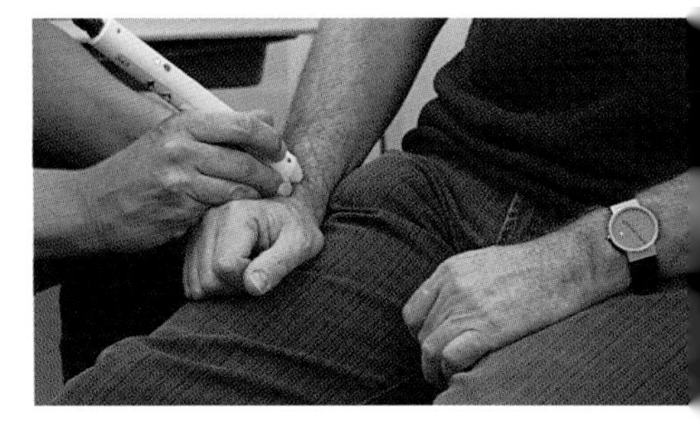

Last but not the least is surgery. Fragment removal, repositioning bones etc can be considered. If medical management fails, then joint replacement surgery may be required.

Joint Replacement

The success story of modern orthopaedic surgery has been with joint replacements. It is the art of replacing painful, arthritic, worn parts with artificial surfaces. These are shaped such so that they allow joint movement.

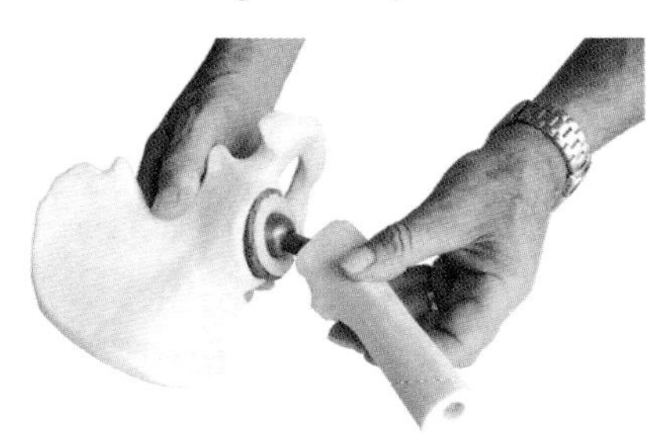

Pre-Operative Planning

The anesthetists do a complete pre-anesthetic work up. As the surgery required is mostly in elderly patients, ECG, X-rays, urine tests, MRI, hematology and biochemistry blood tests are conducted. Cross matching of blood and requirement of blood is also placed with the blood bank. Accurate X-rays of the affected joints are taken and implant design is selected and the size is matched to the X-ray images (i.e. templating).

Post-Operative Rehabilitation

- This involves early mobilization of the patient to reduce the chances of complications, e.g. venous thromboembolism and pneumonia
- Physiotherapy helps the patients recover the joint function after joint replacement surgery
- A planned exercise program is started for the patient The ambulation and motion of the joints is not to be strenuous. Strengthening exercises are recommended after a period of time.

Artificial joints utilize junctions like metal / bone, cement / bone, etc. Ceramic materials are now being offered as new options for joint replacement surgery.

Septic Arthritis

Septic arthritis is also known as infectious arthritis or pyogenic arthritis. Septic arthritis can affect any age group. It occurs when some type of infecting organism, most often bacteria, infects a joint. It is a serious infection of the joints characterized by pain, fever, chills, inflammation and swelling in one or more joints. Septic arthritis can often result in the loss of function of the affected joint. It may result in a medical emergency because it damages the bone as well as cartilage. It can also create a condition for septic shock. Patients receiving corticosteroid injections into the joints for osteoarthritis must be careful of contracting this disease.

Infectious Arthritis

Infectious arthritis results in pain and swelling of the joints (inflammation) and can affect one or more joints. This inflammation can be due to bacterium, a virus or a fungus.

Both men and women can get infected by it. It can affect people of any age.

Individuals more prone to suffer from infectious arthritis are those suffering from :

- Diabetes
- Severe kidney disease
- AIDS
- Any form of immune deficiency
- Any form of cancer
- Alcoholism

Symptoms

- When this disease is caused by a bacterium, the pain and swelling present is only in one spot and can be sudden. It may be accompanied by fever and chills.

- When infectious arthritis is due to viral infection, there may be generalized body pain.
- When the cause is fungal, the pain and swelling develop over a period of time. Mild fever may be present.

Rheumatoid Arthritis (RA)

RA is an autoimmune disease. Rheumatoid arthritis (RA) causes redness, pain, swelling or a hot (or warm) feeling in the lining of a joint (i.e inflammation). The inflammation can affect other internal organs, e.g. eyes, lungs, or heart. The most common areas affected in the body by RA are hands or feet.

Incidence of Rheumatoid Arthritis - Rheumatoid arthritis affects women three times more often than men. Most people develop RA between 25 and 50 years of age.

Symptoms of Rheumatoid Arthritis

- Morning stiffness in joints.
- Pain in three or more joints at the same time.
- Stiffness and swelling in fingers and wrists.
- Pain in the same joints on both sides of the body.
- RA can start gradually or with a sudden, severe attack (flu-like symptoms).
- The disease can be mild showing some periods of activity and joint inflammation.

Diagnosis of Rheumatoid arthritis is by

- Rheumatoid factor determination assay.
- Rheumatoid arthritis specific autoantibodies (Anti CCP)

  RA is more common in the families of people who have this disease. If you are developing RA, then consult your doctor or a rheumatologist.

Foot and Hand Wear

- Avoid wearing tight pointed and uncomfortable footwear (shoes, sandals or chappals). They cause the feet to swell and may lead to bony arthritis.
- Tight socks and stockings which cause toe compression should also be avoided.

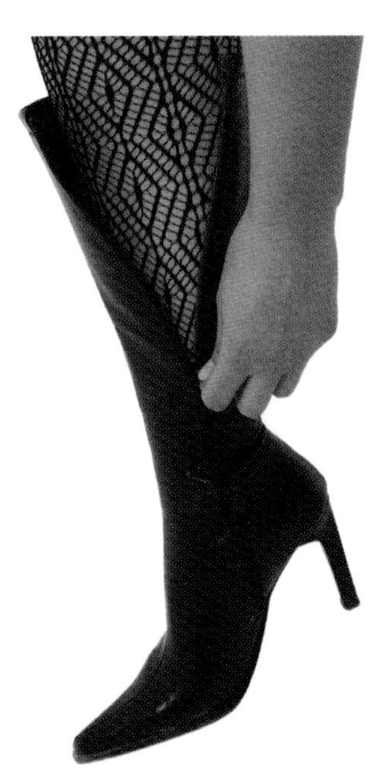

- If out during cold weather wear long warm gloves which protect your wrists from the cold.
- Keep your feet and toes warm with comfortable socks (or wear a double layer of socks).

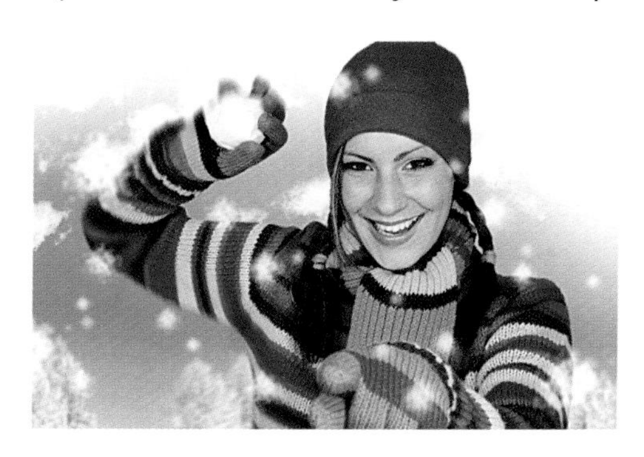

Medication and Diet

Medication given for rheumatoid arthritis tends to 'upset the stomach'. Long term medication can cause gastritis leading to development of gastric ulcer. Spicy and fried food should be avoided. A nutritious balanced diet is recommended (fresh fruits, green vegetables, chicken, lean meats, soya, etc). If an individual is overweight then foods rich in starch should be avoided.

Medicine Normally Prescribed for Rheumatoid Arthritis

- Analgesics
- Disease modifying anti-rheumatic drugs (DMARD's)
- Leflulnomide is a newer class of DMARD for the treatment of rheumatoid arthritis. It helps in reducing tender of swollen joints. It should be taken

only on the advice of your doctor as regular blood counts and other blood tests (hepatotoxicity, etc) must be assayed for side effects.

- Intra-articular corticosteroid injections (to help control exacerbation)

Management of Rheumatoid Arthritis

Rest

Rest is important in rheumatoid arthritis, but correct position while resting is more essential. It is essential to rest most of the time with your legs straight, otherwise, in a few days you will find your legs becoming stiff and fixed in that position. The individual will have to then hobble around.

Resting after a while, should be accompanied by repeated de-freezing exercises. All the joints by turn, should be put through a range of movement every day.

Exercises

Feet and Ankle

Lie down with your legs outstretched. Bend your toes tightly then relax them. Perform this exercise 7 times. For the ankles lie or sit with your knees in a position and move your toes and ankle clockwise and anticlockwise.

Knee

You can lie on your back and perform cycling movements. You can perform “vajarasan” for a minute sitting with your legs under the thighs.

Hips

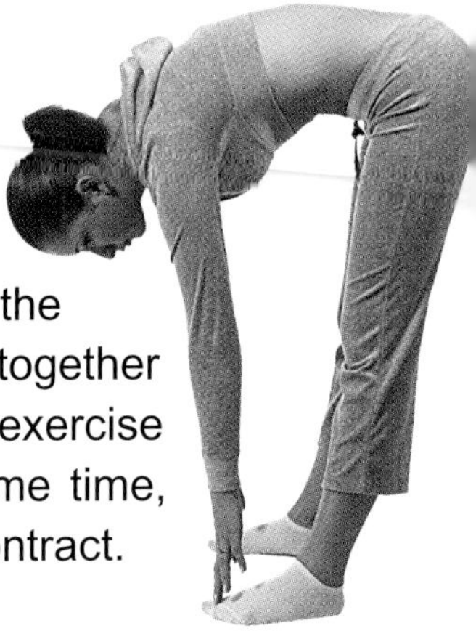

Help rotate the hip joint. Lie on your back, bend both your legs. Then separate both your knees keeping the heels together. Put your knees back together and then straighten your legs. This exercise besides helping rotate the joint same time, prevents the capsule around it to contract.

Spine

Stand up straight and bend forward to touch your toes. Straighten up slowly. Put your hands on your hips and rotate your spine, without moving your feet. Rotate first to right and then to left. Do it a number of times.

Shoulder and Neck

After a day of working on the computer or desk, shoulders become stiff and painful.

- For this shrugging your shoulders up high is a good exercise. Do this 7 times. 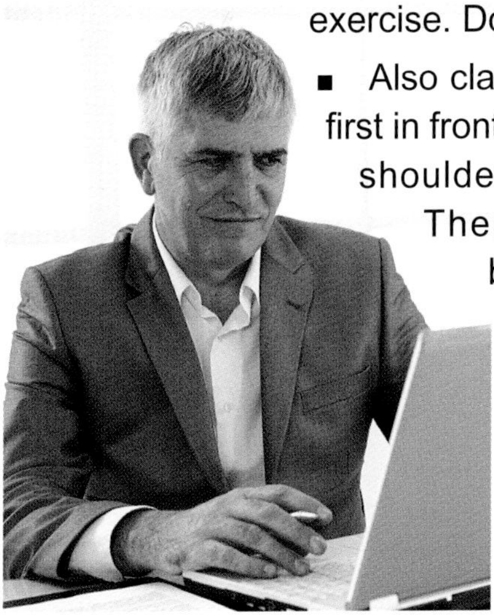
- Also clasp your hands together first in front of your head. Pull your shoulders back and release. Then clasp your hands behind your head and pull your shoulders back and release. Do this exercise 7 times each.

Hands and Fingers

Open your hands and fingers several times and close. Rotate each wrist clockwise and anticlockwise several times a day. For your elbows sit comfortably and stretch your arm as far as you can.

Ankylosing Spondylitis (AS)

Ankylosing spondylitis is arthritis involving the spine and the sacroiliac joints. Men develop it more than women. Often, in women it takes more time to diagnose the disease. AS appears between the ages of 15 years and 40 years. It can start around the knees, hips and, heels. The exact cause of this disease is unknown. It can be present in certain families. It causes pain and stiffness in the back resulting in a bent posture. This is as a result of inflammation in the spinal joints. In severe inflammation the vertebrae can fuse together leading to limited immobility.

Symptoms

- Chronic back pain which lasts for many months or years.
- Back pain that occurs during the night.
- Stiffness in the back in the morning or after periods of rest.
- Recurring inflammation in the eyes causing pain, redness, blurred vision, and sensitivity to bright light.

Treatment

The doctor may ask for X-rays or blood tests like ESR (Erythrocyte Sedimentation Rate) to be done. You may be asked to consult a rheumatologist who will prescribe medications to relieve pain.

Medication

- Non-steroidal anti-inflammatory drugs (NSAIDs)
- Disease-modifying anti-rheumatic drugs (DMARDs) – Patients with severe AS, the drug called sulfasalazine can help manage the symptoms. The most common DMARDs like methotrexate and sulfasalazine are often given along with other medication.
- Corticosteroids - For severe pain and inflammation, cortisone is injected directly into the affected joint.
- Biologics are newer drugs that are becoming available for AS patients that fail to respond to conventional treatment. Biologics are DMARDs which are made up of genetically modified proteins. They work by blocking specific parts of the immune system, called cytokines, which play a role in causing ankylosing spondylitis.

Management of Ankylosing Spondylitis

Exercise

Exercise plays a very important role in managing ankylosing spondylitis. It helps the joints move and reduces pain. Strengthening exercises can be learnt from a physiotherapist. Activities like swimming, and walking can help to keep a good posture. Exercise is also important for maintaining chest expansion.

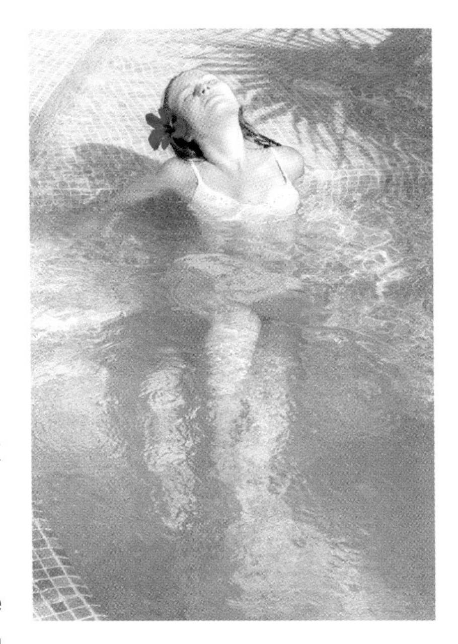

Heat

Heat can help relax aching muscles.

Surgery

In severe or advance cases, ankylosing spondylitis may require surgery for badly damaged joints.

Some other ways for keeping Ankylosis Spondylitis under control are-

- Protect your joints by avoiding excessive mechanical stress from daily tasks.
- Pacing, by alternating heavy or repeated tasks with easier tasks or breaks
- Avoid keeping the joints in the same position for a long time.
- Use a cane or raised chair to help make daily tasks easier and avoid falls.
- Use a firm supportive surface to maintain good spinal alignment.

Spondylitis

Spondylitis is a group of chronic diseases. These diseases primarily affect the spine, although other joints and organs often get involved.

The diseases under spondylitis include:

Psoriatic arthritis: It appears in about 5-10% patients suffering from psoriasis. Psoriasis precedes the arthritic disease.

Reactive arthritis: It is also known as Reiter's Syndrome. It causes inflammation and pain in joints, skin, eyes, bladder, genitals and mucus membranes. This is probably a reaction to the infection which primarily started in some parts of the body.

Juvenile spondyloarthropathy –It is the medical term defining a group of childhood rheumatic diseases. These diseases could continue through adult life also.

Ankylosing spondylitis (AS) – It is a form of chronic autoimmune arthritis. It primarily affects the spine and sacroiliac joints. Other joints often become involved.

Enteropathic arthritis – It is a form of chronic, inflammatory arthritis. It is associated with the presence of an inflammatory bowel disease (IBD) e.g. ulcerative colitis and Crohn's disease.

Pott's disease – It is a form of spondylitis and develops due to the presence of extrapulmonary tuberculosis.

Some Other Painful Ailments

Cervical Spondylosis

Cervical spondylosis is a common disorder of the cervical spine. Degenerative changes in the vertebrae and between the intervertebral discs lead to rheumatoid disease (due to ageing or injury). Compression of the spinal cord occurs due to spondylotic myelopathy which can be present in the advanced stages of this disease.

Symptoms (e.g. pain) are due to

- Osteophytes present on the sides of the vertebrae
- Degeneration of the intervertebral discs
- Changes in the spinal cord and nerves due to insufficient blood supply

Management

- Anti-inflammatory medication, e.g. ibuprofen, piroxicam, aspirin are advised to help relieve pain and swelling.
- Cervical immobilization is done with the help of a collar, etc.
- Studies show that 18% of patients with CSM improve on their own, and stabilize out. It is only 40% that deteriorate without treatment.
- If uncontrollable pain continues or becomes worse, surgical intervention is recommended.

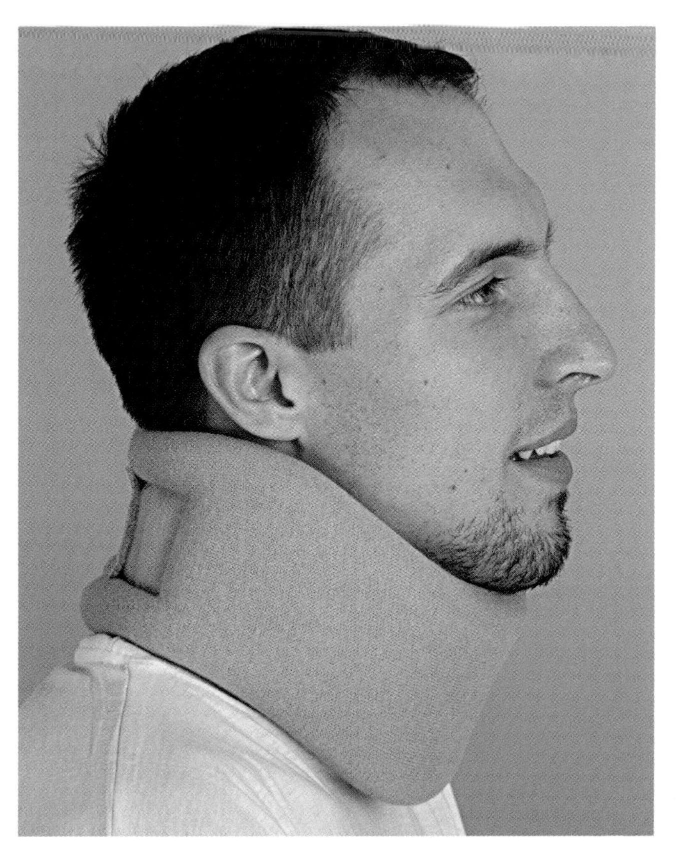

Frozen Shoulder

Frozen shoulder (adhesive capsulitis) is a condition which presents with pain and loss of motion or stiffness in the shoulder. Frozen shoulder often affects individual patients between 40 and 60 years of age. Frozen shoulder is much more common in individuals with diabetes. Increased risk of frozen shoulder also occurs in individuals suffering from diseases like hypothyroidism, hyperthyroidism or Parkinson's disease.

Symptoms

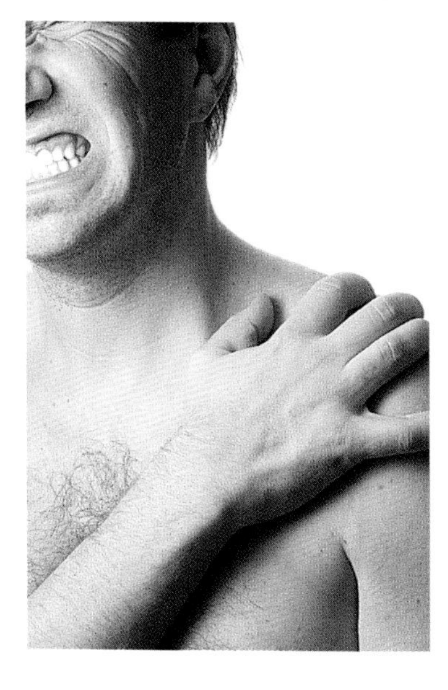

Frozen shoulder pain is dull or aching. It worsens with movement. The pain is usually located over the outer shoulder area and sometimes in the upper arm.

Frozen shoulder first starts with a slow onset of pain. As pain worsens the movement of the shoulder becomes difficult. In the next or 'frozen' stage there is a slow improvement in pain, but the stiffness remains. In the last stage (thawing stage) of frozen shoulder, motion slowly returns towards normal.

X-rays and MRI studies can be performed. Frozen shoulder mostly gets better on its own. It sometimes takes a longer time, recovery occures over two to three years. Pain can be controlled with anti-inflammatory medication. Medical treatment is done through oral medication or by corticosteroid injections. Applying heat or cold compression can also help in pain relief.

Management

Physiotherapy

It includes "stretching or range-of-motion" exercises for the shoulder. If pain is not relieved with time, nerve blocks are sometimes used to subside the pain. More aggressive physical therapy is recommended.

Surgical Treatment

Surgical intervention is considered if there is no improvement in pain or shoulder motion is limited (after an appropriate course of physical therapy and anti-inflammatory medications). In surgical intervention stretching or releasing the contracted joint capsule of the shoulder is done. Shoulder arthroscopy is also an alternative for non-improvement of the disease even after medication. The surgeon makes several small incisions around the shoulder. A small camera and instruments are inserted through the incisions. Tight portions of the joint capsule are cut with the help of the inserted instrument and pressure is relieved. Manipulation can also be done. After surgery, physical therapy is needed to maintain the motion of the shoulder, which was achieved with surgery. Recovery time can take six weeks to three months approximately.

Chronic Back Pain

When an individual experiences pain in any area of the back for a long period of time, he not only suffers the physical aspect but also loses confidence. It this pain remains for a long period of time it is called chronic back pain. The most common area of chronic back injury and pain is the lower back or the lumbar spine.

Common Causes of Chronic Back Pain

- Poor posture - slouching, combined with weak abdominal muscles leads to a swayback, resulting in curving of the spine. This exaggerated curve makes the back ligaments to stretch. Over a period of time the discs between the vertebrae become thin and distorted.
- Frequent cause of back pain is injury due to lifting heavy objects. This can result in straining and disc herniation.
- 80% of back pain is attributed to lack of exercise and poor physical fitness. While lifting heavy objects, strong muscles, especially the abdominal muscles are known to support the back and help distribute weight. Back and abdominal muscles that have lost their flexibility and strength cause more stress on the attached ligaments.
- Certain sports and activities can also be associated with injury and back pain.
- Diseases such as osteoarthritis, ankylosing spondylitis, compression fractures etc., may result in chronic back pain.

- After having performed a physical examination the doctor may recommend X-rays, MRI or other tests to make the diagnosis.
- For relief anti-inflammatory analgesic drugs may be recommended.

The Importance of Exercise in Chronic Back Pain

- Exercise helps reduce pain and prevents further joint damage. It also helps maintain a healthy weight.
- There are different types of exercises:

i) Strengthening exercises: These maintain or increase muscle strength.

ii) Motion exercises: These help to reduce stiffness and keep the joints moving.

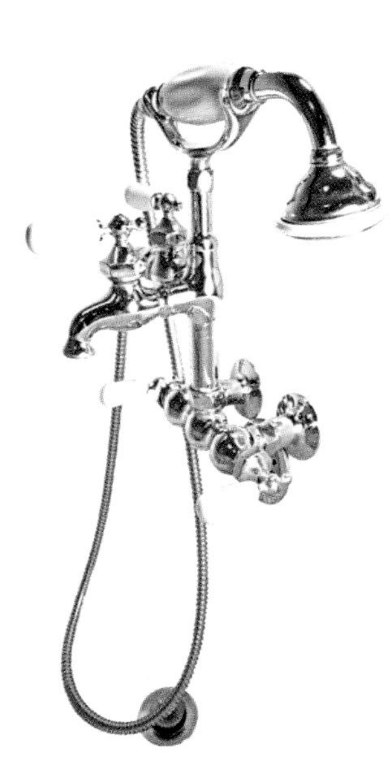

Heat/Cold Compresses

- Applying heat com-pression helps relax aching muscles. It reduces joint pain and soreness. A hot shower is also recommended for the ache.
- Swelling and pain in a joint is relieved by applying a cold pack (ice in a towel).

Prevention

- Be kind to your body. After doing heavy work, slow down by doing an easy task, or take rest.
- When you lift a heavy item keep it as close to your body as possible.
- Maintain a healthy weight and avoid putting extra stress on your joints.
- Be aware of your posture to stand and sit straight.
- Wear proper shoes for walking.
- Sleep on a firm mattress. Do not sleep on your stomach as it can strain your neck.

Relaxation

- Also try and relax the muscles around your joint. Physiotherapy with Ultrasound can help.
- Try deep breathing exercises.

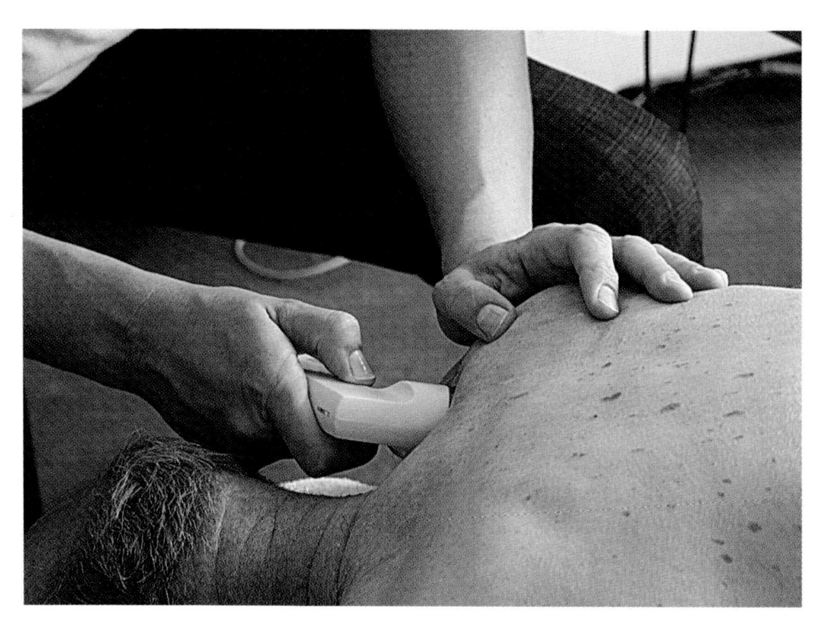

- Listen to music or relaxation tapes.
- Meditate or pray.
- Visualize a pleasant activity like sitting on the beaches.

Surgery

If no medical treatment provides relief, your doctor or rheumatologist may recommend surgery e.g. for a herniated disc.

Gout

Hippocrates described its symptoms 2500 years ago. It has been referred to as a "disease of Kings". Gout is predominantly a disease of adult men who have a higher standard of living. It may be genetic too. Gout occurs mostly in men between 40-50 years of age. The predisposition of this disease is less in women as compared to men.

Gout is an acutely painful disease. The pain is a result of the build up of uric acid crystals in the joints. It most often affects the big toe but also can affect knees, feet, ankles, elbows, wrists and hands.

Gout can be due to the deficiency of Hypoxanthine-Guanine Phosphoribosyl Transferase (HGPRT). The feedback to inhibit uric acid production is less so that more of uric acid is produced (Uric acid is a natural waste product of the body, which is excreted by the kidneys). Gout is a case of excessive uric acid production or not enough excretion. The uric acid formed into crystals deposits into the joints (urate) causing swelling, pain and tenderness in the affected area.

Other causes of excessive uric acid production can be due to certain medication like low dose aspirin and thiazide diuretics. These interfere with uric acid excretion by the kidneys. Hyperuricemia (or excessive uric acid production) can be due to secondary causes as well.

Remember

- Fresh fruits and vegetables help to reduce uric acid levels.

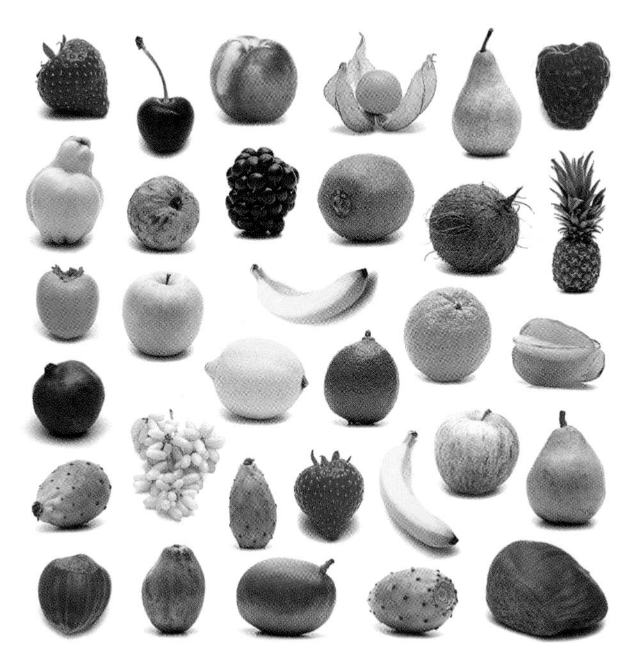

- Medication like allopurinol, corticosteroids, or colchicine can be recommended by the doctor for treating gout.
- Strengthening exercises must be done to increase the muscle strength of the affected joints.

- Avoid high uric acid and non-vegetarian foods, e.g. kidney, liver, brain, gravies, and alcoholic drinks like red wine, port, heavy beers and Champagne.

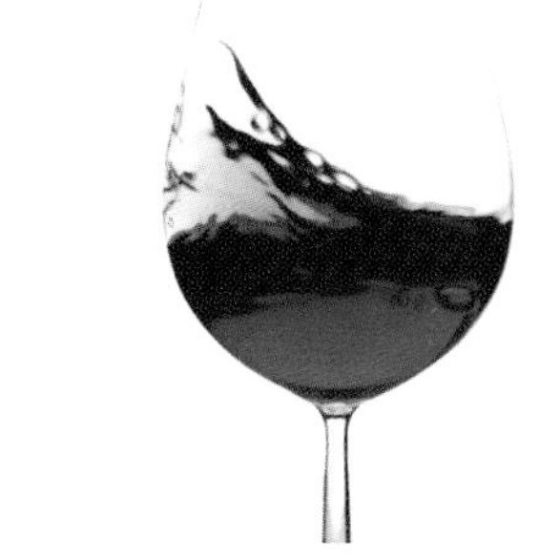

Myalgia

Myalgia means 'muscle pain'. It is the cause of many diseases. The most common causes of myalgia are overuse, injury or stress of muscles. Myalgia can also be caused due to certain medication, as a response to vaccination and withdrawal syndromes (e.g. alcohol or barbiturate withdrawal).

For muscle pain from overuse or injury, take acetaminophen or ibuprofen. Apply ice for the first 24 to 72 hours of an injury to reduce pain and inflammation.

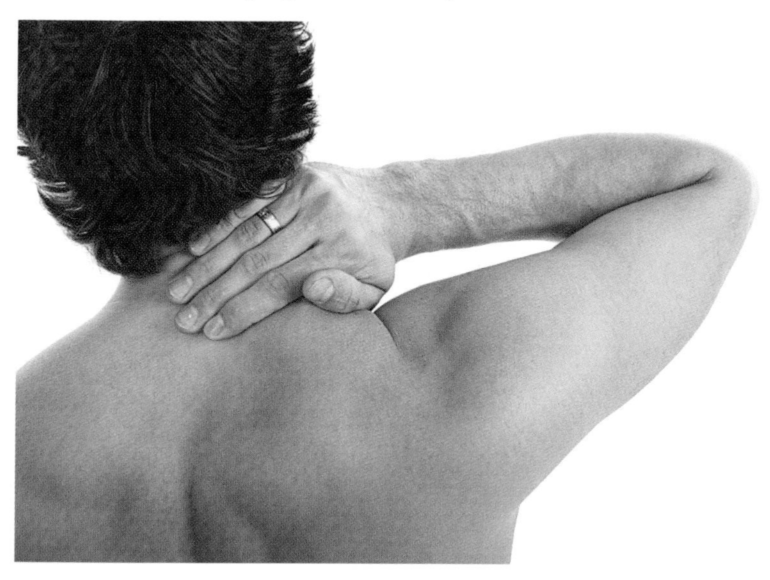

Later, heat application on the affected site often feels more soothing. Muscle aches from overuse and fibromyalgia often respond well to massage. Regular exercise can help restore proper muscle tone. High-impact aerobic activities should be avoided when injured or while in pain. Plenty of sleep and reducing your stress help. If home remedies don't work, visit your doctor. He may consider medication, physical therapy referral, or referral to a specialised pain clinic. If your muscle aches are due to a specific disease, follow your doctor's advice and treat the primary illness.

Consult a doctor if:

- Your muscle pain persists beyond 2 days
- You have severe, unexplained pain
- You have any sign like swelling or redness around the tender muscle
- You have poor circulation in the area where you have muscle aches (for example, in your legs).

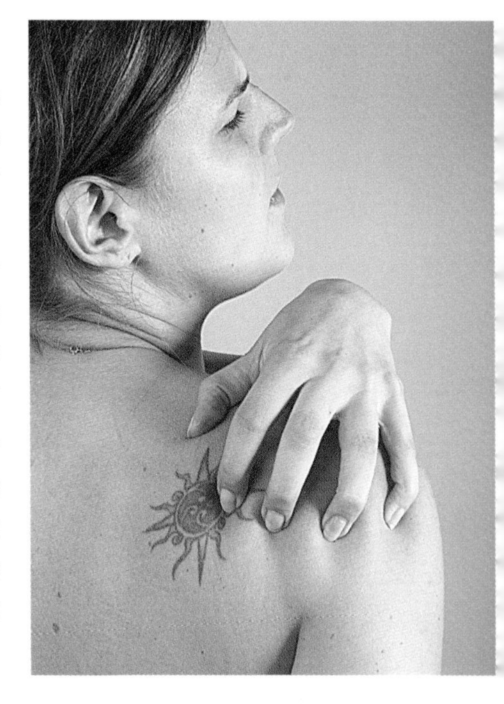

Your muscle pain has been associated with starting or changing doses of a medicine, such as a statin.

Osteoporosis is more common in women but can also develop in elderly men. It occurs due to hormonal disorders, chronic diseases and as a side effect of medication (like glucocorticoids).

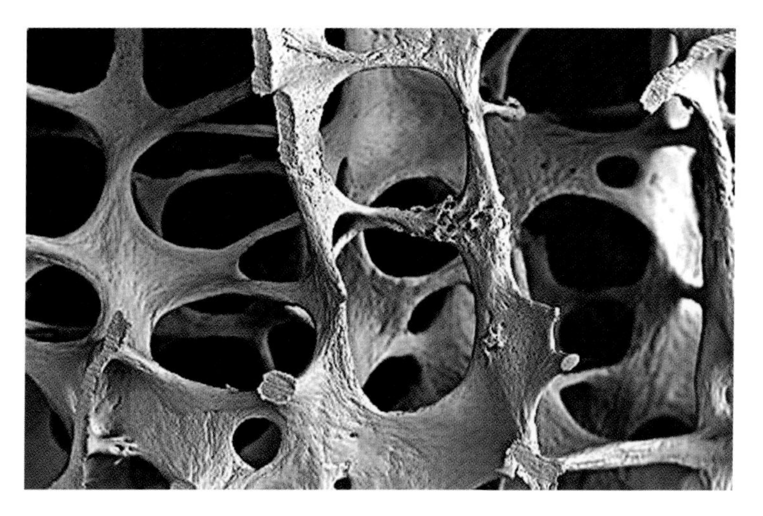

Fractures due to Osteoporosis

Vertebral collapse or ('compression fracture') is observed with sudden back pain in osteoporosis. Multiple vertebral fractures often lead to a stooped posture, loss of height, and chronic pain. Fractures of the long bones can impair mobility and may require surgery. Hip fracture requires prompt surgery, as complications such as deep vein thrombosis and pulmonary embolism can occur.

Risk of Fall

An increased risk, to a person in the geriatric age group. The individual's fall can lead to fractures of the wrist, spine or hip. Causes of falling are many, e.g. irregular heartbeat, vasovagal syncope, etc. Removal of obstacles like loose carpets, slippery tiles or granite in the bathroom may substantially reduce slipping and falling.

Diagnosis

The diagnosis of osteoporosis is made by measuring the bone mineral density (BMD).

X-ray absorptiometry (DXA or DEXA) is the usual method. Also blood tests and X-rays if required may be conducted on the patient.

Risks Leading to Osteoporosis

Non-modifiable Risks

- Estrogen deficiency in women following menopause.
- Family history of osteoporosis
- There are at least 30 known genes associated with the development of osteoporosis.

Modifiable Risks

- Vitamin D deficiency: Mild vitamin D insufficiency is seen to increase with Parathyroid Hormone (PTH) production. PTH increases bone reabsorption, leading to bone loss.

- Calcium – low levels of calcium and decreased protein intake is associated with lower peak bone mass during adolescence. Lower bone mineral density was observed in elderly individuals.
- Excess alcohol – heavy drinking (intake greater than 2 units/day) increases the risk for developing osteoporosis.
- Tobacco smoking - tobacco smoking inhibits the activity of osteoblasts. It is an independent risk factor for developing osteoporosis.
- Weight bearing exercise helps increase peak bone mass. Physical inactivity leads to significant bone loss.

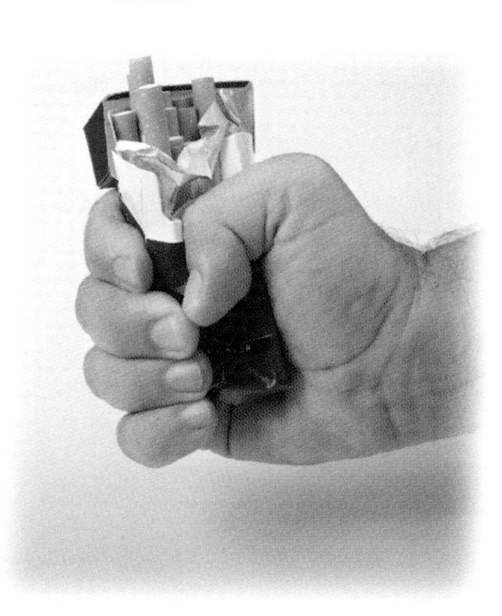

- Excess physical activity on the other hand leads to constant damages of various parts of the body (e.g. ligaments, joints, etc). In women, heavy exercise can lead to decreased estrogen levels, pre-disposing them to osteoporosis.

- Heavy metals, eg. cadmium often leads to loss of bone mineral density leading to pain and increased risk of fractures.

Secondary Osteoporosis

Causes

- Hypogonadal states, e.g Turner syndrome
- A bilateral oophorectomy (surgical removal of the ovaries) or deficient estrogen production. In males, testosterone deficiency is the cause.
- Common endocrine disorders causing bone loss can be due to hyperparathyroidism, thyrotoxicosis, hypothyroidism, diabetes mellitus type 1 and 2, adrenal insufficiency, etc.
- Malnutrition, parenteral nutrition and malabsorption can lead to osteoporosis. Certain gastrointestinal disorders (e.g. coeliac disease) predispose an individual to osteoporosis,.
- Rheumatologic disorders like rheumatoid arthritis, ankylosing spondylitis, etc can lead to osteoporosis.
- Hematologic disorders, e.g. multiple myeloma are also linked to osteoporosis.

Modicatlon

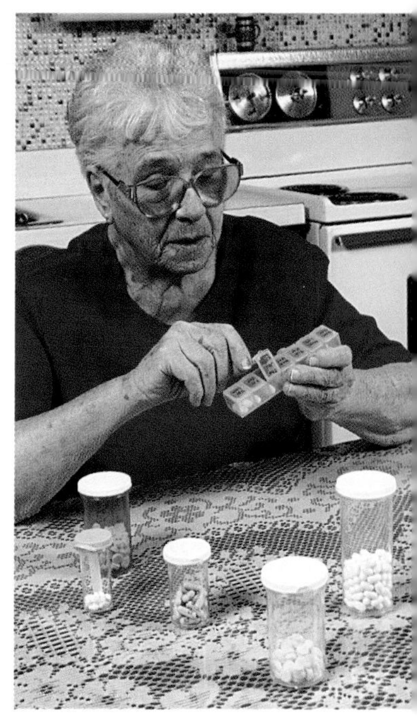

Medication which can be associated with an increase in osteoporosis are :

- Anticoagulants and warfarin. Long-term use of heparin is also associated with a decrease in bone density.
- Proton pump inhibitors inhibit the production of stomach acid. They also interfere with calcium absorption (e.g. rabe-prazole, omeprazole).

Thiazolidinedione (used for diabetes) e.g. rosiglitazone has been linked to an increased risk of osteoporosis and fracture.

Role of Calcium and Magnesium in Preventing Bone Loss

- Magnesium is a mineral which helps in maintaining healthy bones. It contributes to increased bone density and helps prevent the onset of osteoporosis.
- Magnesium helps the body absorb calcium.
- Osteoclasts and osteoblasts are stimulated by hormones like parathyroid hormone (PTH) and calcitonin. PTH makes the osteoclasts deplete calcium from the bones,

- Lack of magnesium causes imbalance between PTH and calcitonin resulting in bone loss. Magnesium supplementation helps correct this process.
- Large amounts of processed food deplete magnesium from the diet.
- A 2:1 calcium-to-magnesium ratio is required for an individual.
- Lack of calcium and magnesium may cause leg cramps during the night.
- Also for maximum absorption of magnesium, calcium supplements should be taken.

Osteopenia

Osteopenia is bone mineral density (BMD) which is lower than normal peak BMD.

As one advances with age, bones start losing minerals, heaviness (mass), and structure. This makes the bones weaker and increases their risk of breaking. Individuals begin losing bone mass after about 30 years of age.

Some people having osteopenia may not have bone loss. They just have a natural lower bone density. Women are more likely to develop osteopenia due to a lower peak BMD. The loss of bone mass increases with hormonal changes, especially during perimenopausal or menopausal stage.

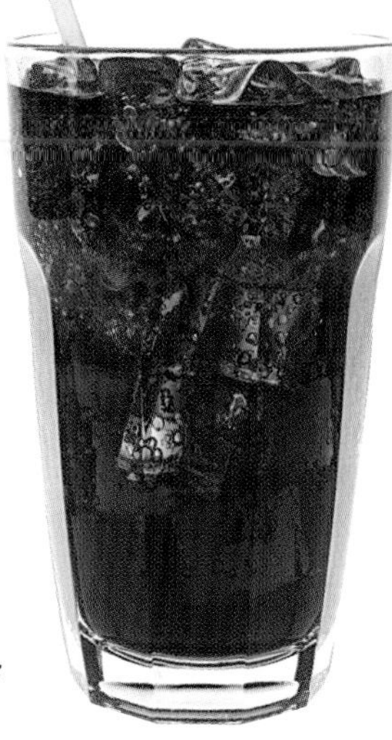

Causes

- Eating disorders or metabolic problems
- Chemotherapy, or medications (e.g. steroids)
- Exposure to radiation
- Family history of osteoporosis
- Taking aerated drinks or alcohol excessively increases the risk of osteopenia.

Treatment of Osteoporosis and Osteopenia

- Lifestyle changes
- Calcium supplements combined with vitamin D should be taken. Vitamin D helps the body absorb calcium and other minerals. Vitamin D is present in, eggs, salmon, sardines, swordfish and some fish oils. Calcium is present in milk and milk products.
- Exercise is important in maintaining strong bones. Weight-bearing exercises such as walking, hiking, and dancing are all good choices. Adding exercise with light weights or elastic bands can help bones in the upper part of the body.

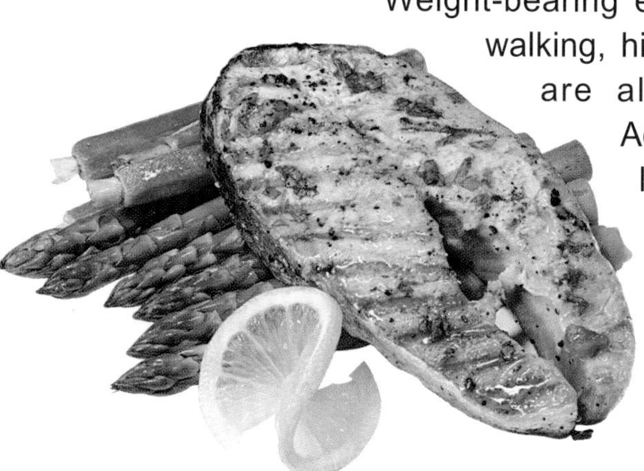

Osteomalacia

Osteomalacia results in softening of the bones due to defective bone mineralization. Osteomalacia is specifically a defect in mineralization of the protein framework known as osteiod. Osteomalacia is derived from the Greek word '*osteo*' referring to bone and '*malacia*' means softness.

Symptoms

Diffuse body pains

Muscle weakness

Fragility of the bones

Causes

- Deficiency in Vitamin D (which is obtained from the diet and/or sunlight exposure) especially in dark-skinned individuals.
- Faulty metabolism of Vitamin D or phosphorus
- Renal tubular acidosis
- Malnutrition during pregnancy
- Malabsorption syndrome
- Chronic renal failure

Treatment

Administration of 200,000 IU weekly of vitamin D for 4 to 6 weeks, followed by a maintenance dose of 1600 IU daily or 200,000 IU every 4 to 6 months.

Laboratory Values

Alk.phosphatase	33 – 131 IU/L
Calcium	8.8 – 10.3 mg/dl
Phosphorus	2.50 – 4.6 mg/dl
25OH$_3$ Vitamin D	7.600 – 75.00 ng/ml

Rickets

Rickets leads to fractures and deformity due to softening of bones in children. The predominant cause of rickets is deficiency of Vitamin D. Lack of adequate calcium in the diet may also lead to rickets.

Children at higher risk for developing rickets include

- Breast-fed infants whose mothers are not exposed to sunlight.
- Breast-fed infants not exposed to enough sunlight.
- Children consuming fortified milk due to lactose intolerance.

Symptoms of Rickets

- Pain in the bones or tenderness
- Dental problems
- Muscle weakness

- Increased tendency of fractures
- Skeletal deformity, bowed legs, knock-knees, cranial, spinal, and pelvic deformities
- Tetany
- Craniotabes (soft skull)
- Costochondral swelling ('rickety rosary')

Diagnosis

Blood tests: Serum calcium may show low levels of calcium and serum phosphorus. Serum alkaline phosphatase levels may be high.

X-ray: X-ray of affected bones may show a loss of calcium from bones or a change in the shape of structure of the bones.

Treatment and prevention of rickets : -

- Increased dietary intake of calcium, phosphates and vitamin D (ultraviolet light), along with cod liver oil, halibut-liver oil, and viosterol.
- Ultraviolet in the sunlight each day and adequate supplies of calcium and phosphorus in the diet can prevent rickets. Darker-skinned babies should be exposed longer to the ultraviolet rays. Recommendations are for 200 international units (IU) of vitamin D a day for infants and children.

Role of Vitamins

Vitamin D deficiency leads to rickets in children and osteomalacia in adults. Vitamin D is mostly obtained from the action of ultra-violet light on the skin. Vitamin

D is hydrozylated by the kidney to its active form. On diagnosis of either rickets or osteomalacia, a dose of intra muscular vitamin D is given followed by regular oral supplementation.

Natural Sources of Vitamin D

- Fish liver oils, such as cod liver oil, 1 tbs. (15 ml) provides 1,360 IU
- Fatty fish e.g.
- Salmon (cooked) – 3.5 oz provides 360 IU
- Herring – 85 gm (3 oz) provides 1383 IU
- Sardines (canned in oil), drained – 1.75 oz, 250 IU
- Tuna (canned in oil) – 3 oz, 200 IU
- Mackerel (cooked) – 3.5 oz, 345 IU
- Mushroom provided over 2700 IU per serving (approx ½ cup) of vitamin D, if exposed to just 5 minutes of UV light after being harvested.
- One whole egg, 20 IU

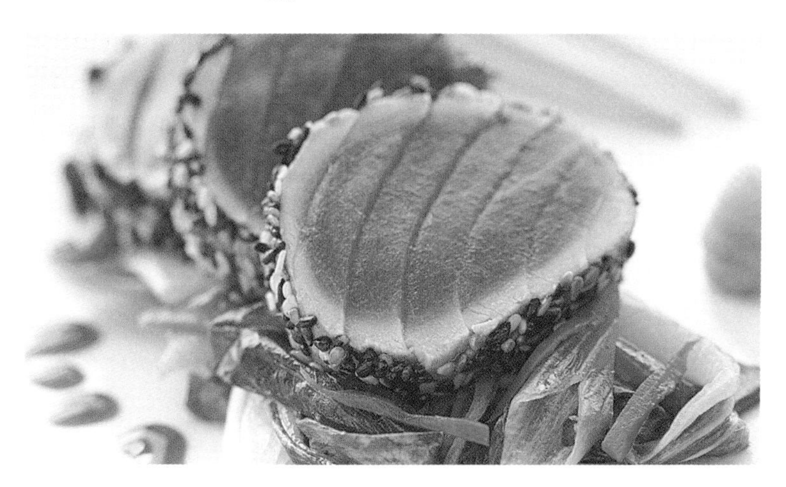

Note: In the major dietary sources of vitamin D, only fish is naturally rich in vitamin D.

Other sources of vitamin D are fortified foods like breakfast cereals, vitamin D supplements and soya milk.

Recommended Dietary Allowance (RDA)

- **Vitamin D**: RDA - 200 international units for most individuals; 400 IUs for people from 51 to 70 years of age.
- **Vitamin E**: RDA - 15 milligrams. Upper limit - 600 milligrams. High levels of vitamin E can cause bleeding.
- **Calcium**: RDA for most adults - 1,000 milligrams daily; for teenagers - 1,200 milligrams; for individuals above the age of 50 - 1,000 milligrams. The richest sources of calcium are dairy and calcium-fortified orange juice.
- **Protein**: An individual should increase his content of protein to about 60 mg/day. It helps in repairing of cells and tissues. Proteins are available in most animal foods like eggs, meat, poultry, fish. In vegetarain foods, diary products, legumes, nuts and beans have a good protein content.

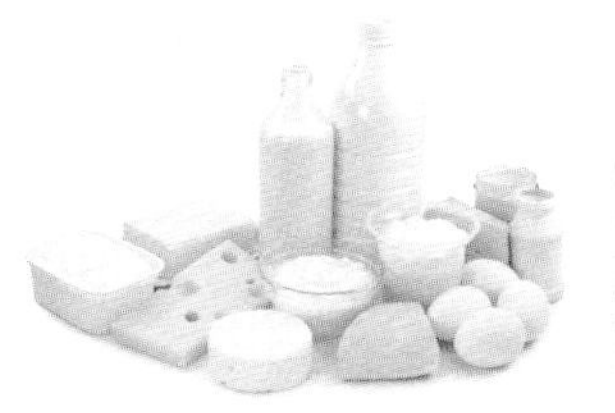

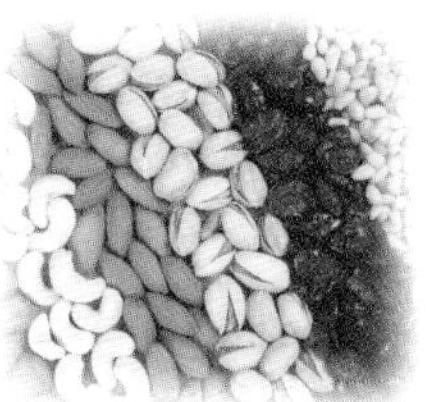

3 Sports Injuries

A sports injury is related to an injury occuring during a sports activity. Injuries often result from accidents, e.g. two sportsmen colliding during a game, use of improper exercising equipment, or insufficient warm up and stretching. Any part of the body can be affected during any sports activity or exercise. Sports injury normally involves the musculoskeletal system (which includes the muscles, bones, and associated tissues like cartilage).

Common Types of Sports Injuries

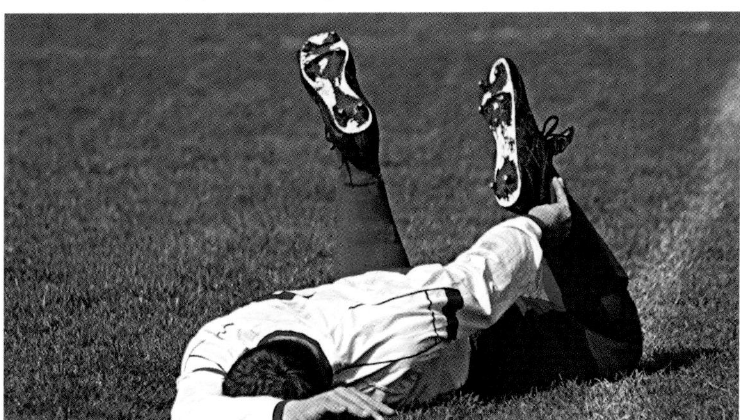

- Muscle sprains and strains
- Ligament Tears
- Tears of the tendons that support joints and allow them to move
- Fractured bones, including vertebrae

- Dislocated joints
- Sprains and Strains

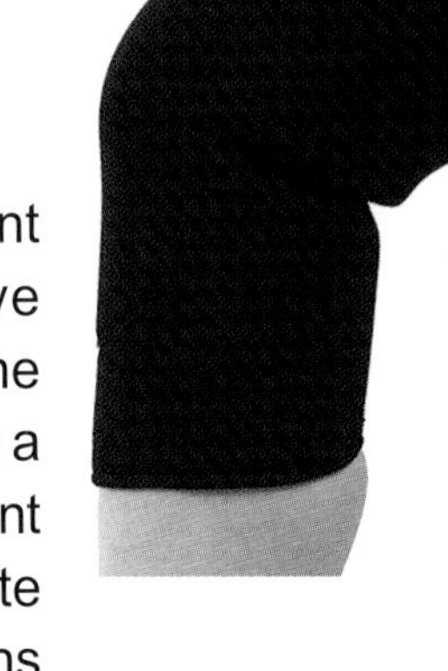

Sprain

Sprain is a stretch or tear of a ligament (ligament is the band of connective tissues that joins one end of the bone with another). Sprains can range from a first-degree minimally stretched ligament (to a third degree tear), i.e. a complete tear). Areas most vulnerable to sprains are ankles, knees, and wrists. Signs of a sprain involve pain, bruising, inflammation, inability to move a limb or joint and instability of the affected part.

Strain

Strain is a twist, pull, or tear of a muscle or tendon (a cord of tissue connecting muscle to bone). Symptoms of a strain include pain, muscle spasm, and loss of strength. Severe strains not treated professionally often cause damage and loss of function.

Achilles Tendon Injury

This injury is caused when the tendon connecting the calf muscle to the back of the heel is stretched or torn. This can occur suddenly and is extremely painful. The most common cause of Achilles tendon

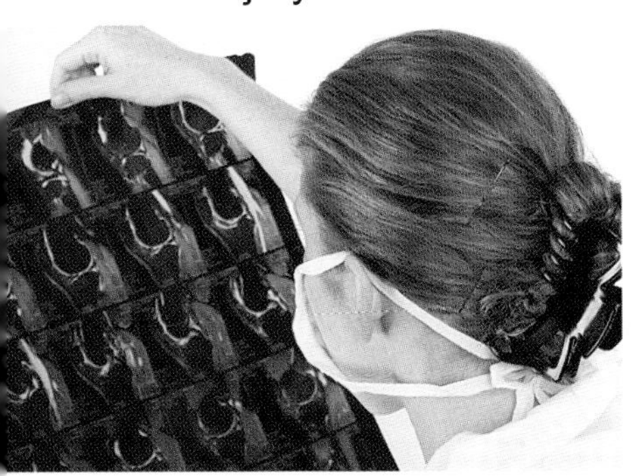

tear is called tendonitis (a degenerative condition caused by overuse or aging).

Fracture

A fracture is a break in the bone. It can be a one-time injury or repeated stress to the bone over time leading to a stress fracture.

- **Acute fracture**: Acute fracture can be simple, i.e. clean break with little damage to the surrounding tissues.
- **Compound fracture:** It is a break in which the bone pierces the skin.

Dislocations

Separation of two bones which form a joint leads to dislocation. Majority of dislocations occur in contact sports such as football and basketball. High-impact sports lead to excessive stretching or falling can also result in dislocation of a joint. A dislocated joint requires immediate medical treatment. The most likely dislocated joints are those of the hands and shoulders.

Acute and Chronic Injuries

Acute Injuries – A sprained ankle or a fractured hand, on activity, is classified under an acute injury. It can result in

- Swelling
- Sudden and severe pain
- Inability to move a joint through its full range of motion
- Visible dislocation or breaking of a bone

Chronic Injuries - Chronic injuries result from overusing a particular area of the body over a long period of time. Chronic injury results in:

- Pain on activity
- A dull ache when resting
- Swelling of the area affected

Advice on Injury

- Work out should not be done during the phase of acute injury or severe pain.
- Rest- Reduce your regular exercise or activities, till the pain subsides.
- Ice -An ice pack should be applied to the injured site for about 20 minutes at a time. It can be done four to eight times a day. A cold pack or ice bag with crushed ice wrapped in a towel can be used. Do not apply the ice for more than 20 minutes, as it can result in cold injury.
- Compression- Compression of the injured area helps reduce swelling and splints.
- To provide support, a splint can be attached to the injured area.
- Ask your doctor for advice, on the type of split to be used.

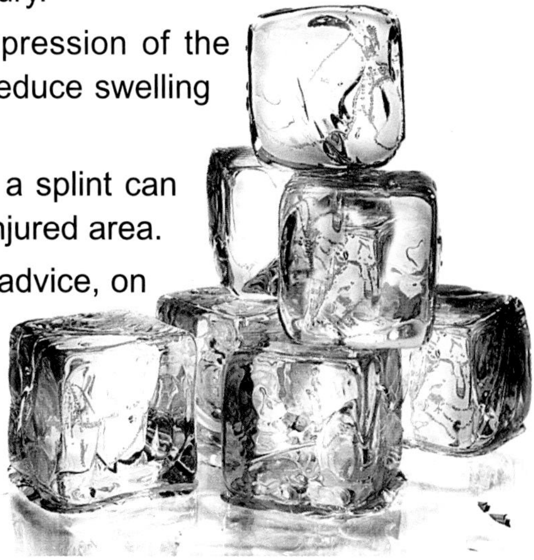

- Elevation - If possible, keep the injured part e.g. ankle, knee, elbow, or wrist elevated on a pillow. It should be placed above the level of the heart, to help decrease the swelling.

Caution

Do not use heat immediately after an injury. This tends to increase the internal bleeding or swelling. Heat is used later to relieve muscle tension and promote relaxation.

Treatment

- Non-steroidal Anti-Inflammatory Drugs (NSAIDs) to reduce inflammation and pain
- Immobilization
- Sling to immobilise the arm, shoulder.
- Splint and cast to support and protect injured bone and soft tissues.
- Leg immobiliser to keep the knee from bending after injury or surgery.
- Surgery - Surgery may be needed to repair torn connective tissue. A Compound fracture may also be realigned. Often, many types of sports injury do not require surgery.

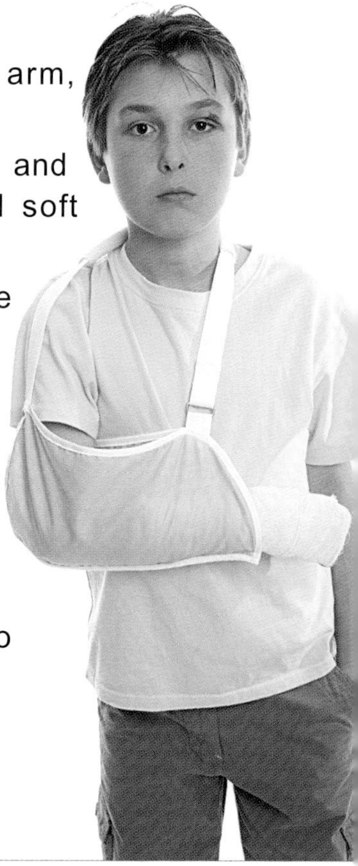

- Rehabilitation - After a sports injury, repair and early mobilisation is seen to speed up healing. Mobilisation can be with gentle stretching and strengthening exercises. Slowly weights may be added to your exercise routine.

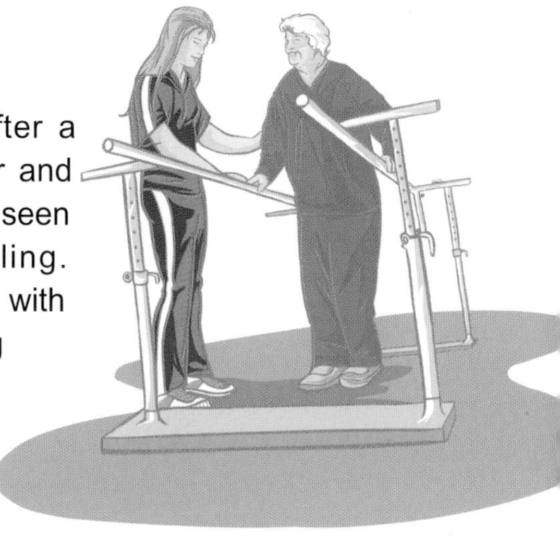

Common Sports Injuries

Badminton Injuries

- Ankle Sprain
- Muscle strain
- Meniscus Tear

Other injuries

- Lateral epicondylitis (Tennis Elbow)
- Medial Epicondylitis (Golfer's Elbow)

  In any sport, a chronic degenerative change of the Achilles tendon can occur due to repetitive jumping, poor recovery, warm up and stretching.

Cramps – occur as sudden, tight and intense pain by a group of muscle locked in spasm. This can be due to excessive fluid loss, excessive heat gain, fatigue and inadequate muscle recovery.

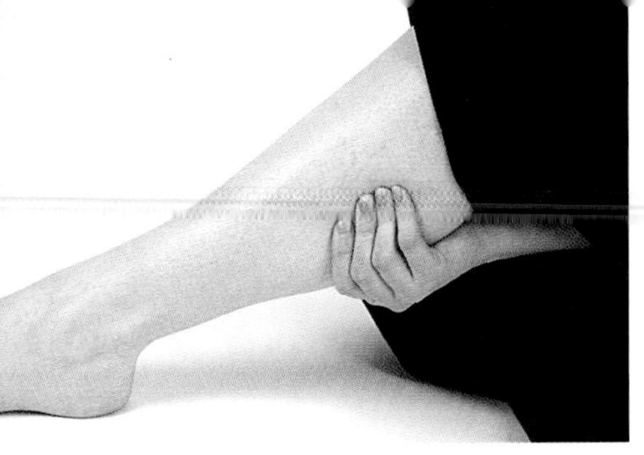

Blisters – Occur mostly on the heels and toes or the hand. They are fluid filled space under the skin caused by direct contact with a hard surface.

Repetitive Stress Injury

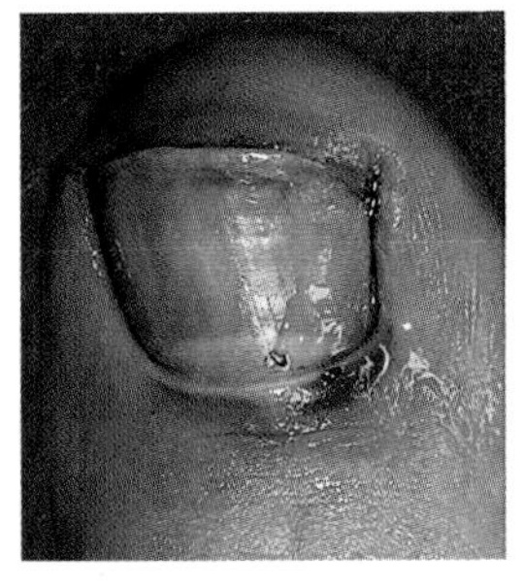

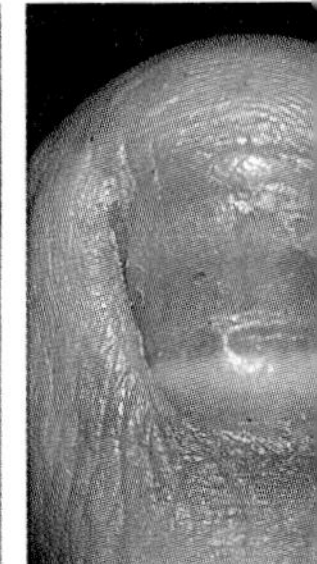

Repetitive stress injury is the name given to a group of conditions that are caused when too much stress is placed on a joint. Repetitive stress injury occurs when the same action is performed over and over again. It can cause pain and swelling in the affected are as muscles, tendons and bursae. Tendons are the strong flexible bands of tissue that attach muscles to the bones. Bursae are small sacs filled with fluid that act as cushions between tendons and bones. The common types of repetitive stress injury are tendinitis and bursitis (inflammation of bursa). Repetitive stress injury generally occurs in those over the age of 30. This is due to the normal wear and tear of aging. It can also occur more frequently in those participating in sports activities.

Signs of repetitive stress injury

- **Pain in a specific area**

  The affected area becomes inflamed, tender and swollen.

Specific types of repetitive stress are:

- **Tennis elbow**

  It is an inflammation of the muscles attached to the outside of the elbow.

- **Golfer's elbow**

  It is an inflammation of the muscles on the inside of the elbow.

- **Trigger finger**

  It is an inflammation of the tendons in your hand (these tendons help you use make a fist).

- **Housemaid's knee**

  It is an inflammation of the bursa on the front of the kneecap.

Remedy

A physical examination of the area is performed by the doctor to confirm the diagnosis.

Medication

Non-steroidal anti-inflammatory drugs. Sometimes cortisone is prescribed, if the swelling persists.

Knee Ligament Injuries

The knee is the weight bearing joint of the body. Its stability depends upon the ligaments and muscles around it. The knee has two important sets of ligaments – the cruciate ligaments and the collateral ligaments.

The Cruciate Ligaments

The cruciate ligaments are present within the knee joint. They are connected from the thighbone (femur) to the shinbone (tibia). They help to hold the bones of the knee joint tightly together, when the leg is bent or straight. This aids in proper knee joint movement. The cruciate ligaments cross each other to form an 'X' . The term cruciate is derived from the Latin word crux, which means 'cross.'

Anterior Cruciate Ligament Injury

Causes

- Changing direction rapidly
- Direct collision, e.g. in football play
- Landing from a jump

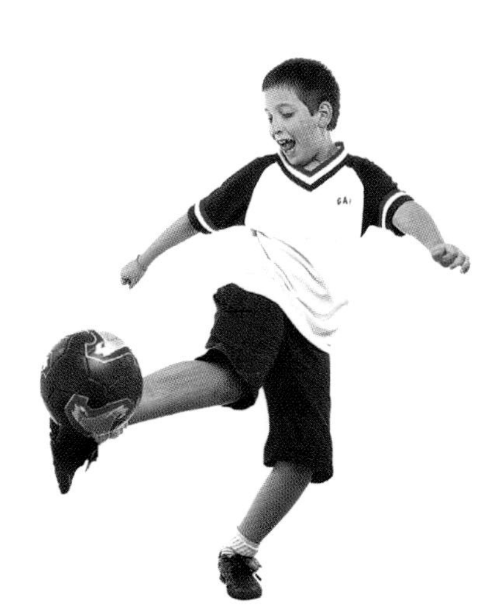

Diagnosis

Your doctor will order an X-ray MRI (Magnetic Resonance Imaging) of the knee joint.

Treatment

- **Non-surgical treatment** – Muscle strengthening along with the use of a brace to provide stability. Activities will be limited for a period of time.
- **Surgical Treatment** – Arthroscopic surgery or open surgery may be performed.

Posterior Cruciate Ligament Injury

Causes

- Blow to the front of the knee
- Pulling or stretching of the ligament

  Diagnosis will be done after the doctor has seen your X-ray and a MRI. In most patients not having symptoms of knee instability, surgery is not required.

Collateral Ligament Injury

The collateral ligaments are situated on the inner and outer side of the knee joint. They provide stability to the knee joint. The injury to the inner or medial collateral ligament usually occurs due to impact on the outside of the knee. It is often accompanied by a sharp pain inside the knee.

Treatment

- Rest
- Putting ice packs on the knee joint
- You may have to wear a bandage for a while
- Elevate the knee whenever possible
- Rehabilitation exercises for good healing should be done.

Colles Fracture

A colles fracture is break across the end of the radius, (or distal fracture) with dorsal (posture) displacement of the wrist. The radius is the long bone of the forearm.

Cause

The primary cause of the colles fracture is due to a fall. The impact of the fall and bodyweight cause the radius to buckle through injury and break. Fall in the elderly often leads to a colles fracture.

Treatment

- An ice pack is put on the wrist to reduce the swelling.
- The wrist is elevated and placed in a sling.

  Consult the Orthopaedician

X-rays and casting of the wrist can be recommended by your orthopaedician. A cast is put on the affected area. Rehabilitation is to continue range of movement in the fingers, thumb and shoulder on the side of the affected wrist. This will help prevent stiffness in these areas. The plaster is normally removed after 6 weeks of injury. This will be after your orthopaedician has had a look at your X-ray.

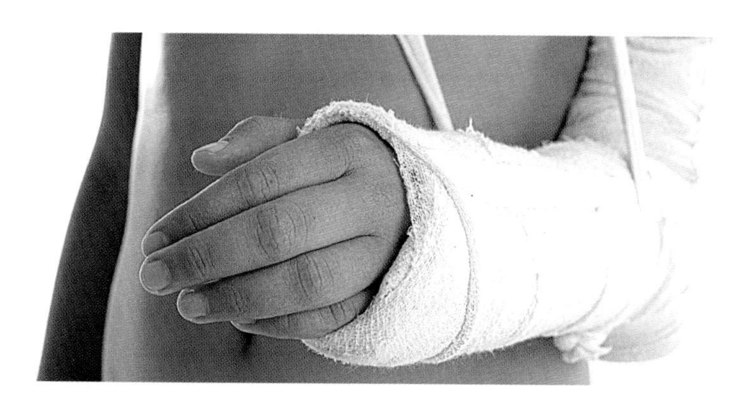

4 Physiotherapy and Acupuncture

Physiotherapy helps the individual (suffering from injury, disease or age) restore maximum movement and functional ability through life. Physiotherapy is associated with some specialities like cardiopulmonary, orthopaedic, neurology and pediatrics. Patient rehabilitation facilities can be available with education and research centres, schools, hospitals, industrial workplaces, fitness and sports centres and some homes.

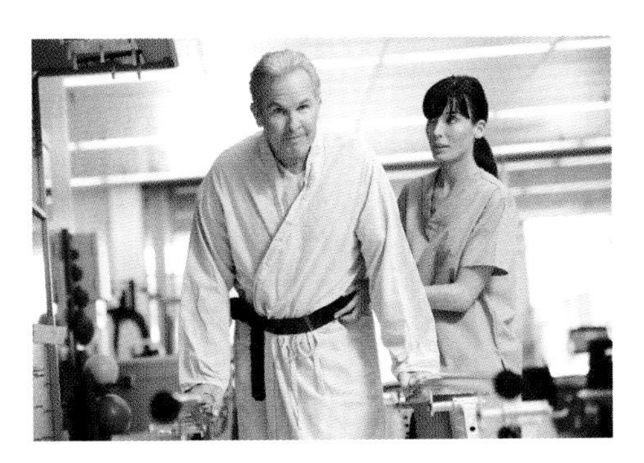

Specialities

Cardiopulmonary

Cardiovascular and pulmonary rehabilitation deals with clearing of lung secretions, e.g in cystic fibrosis, heart attacks, post coronary bypass surgery and chronic obstructive pulmonary disease to name a few. Treatment can benefit much from cardiovascular and pulmonary physical therapy.

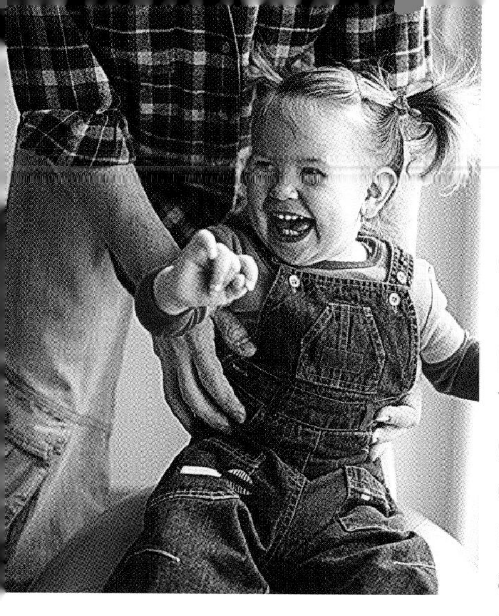

Pediatric

Children with cerebral palsy, spina bifida, developmental delays are treated by physiotherapists. Treatment focusing on modalities like gross and fine motor skills, coordination, strength, cognitive and sensory perceptions are helped by the pediatric therapists.

Orthopaedic

Orthopaedic therapists diagnose, manage and treat disorders and injuries of the musculoskeletal system. Orthopaedic therapists help to treat fractures, acute sport injuries, arthritis, sprains, post-operative orthopaedic procedures etc. Therapeutic exercises, hot and cold packs, electrical stimulation, manipulation are part of their operational procedure.

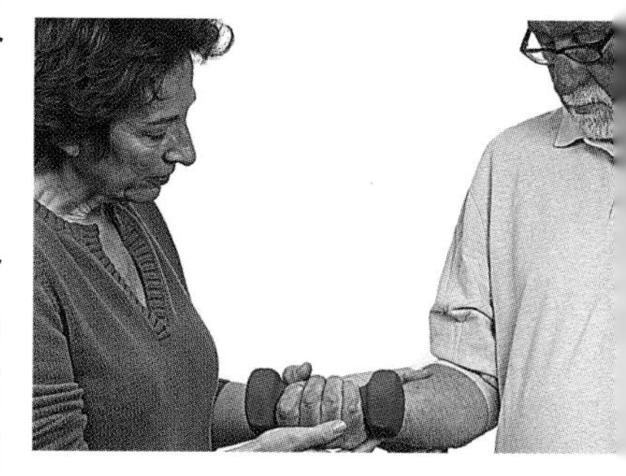

Neurological

Neurological disorders or diseases including Alzheimer's disease, brain injury, cerebral palsy, multiple sclerosis and Parkinson's disease are some of the ailments treated by a neurological therapist. These therapists help their patients to improve these areas of dysfunction.

Geriatric

Geriatric physiotherapy helps the normal ageing adult. Maladies like arthritis, osteoporosis, cancer, Alzheimer's disease, joint replacement, balance disorders, etc are looked after in this group. The aim here is to help restore mobility, reduce pain, and increase fitness level.

Acupuncture

Acupuncture is derived from the Latin word Acuspungere, Acus meaning 'needle', and pungere, 'prick'. World health organization (WHO) comments that this procedure is safe, but needs more research. It is a technique of inserting and manupulating fine filliform needles into specific points on the body. The aim of this technique is to relieve pain and be used for therapeutic purposes. Accupuncture is described in the traditonal Chinese medical texts, as pathways through which Qi and "Blood" flow. Treatment of acupuncture points are performed along several layers of pathways throughout the body (tweleve primary channels or mai). The points to be treated by the acupuncturist are decided after tallying and observation of detailed history of the patient.

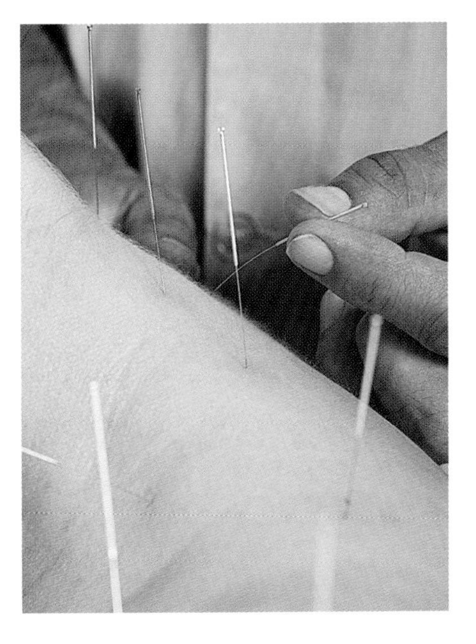

5 Different Sensations of Pain

Earache

Earache is a common medical problem occuring both in children and adults. Common conditions causing earache can be infection of the outer ear (otitis externa) and infection of the middle ear (otitis media).

Otitis externa – It is the infection of the outer ear or ear canal. It often occurs after swimming. Earache can be severe. Mild cases present with an itch more than the pain. There can be hearing loss, ringing or buzzing sounds in the ear and swelling of the ear.

Otitis media- It leads to an infection of the middle ear and eardrum. This occurs due to bacteria growing in the middle ear. Presentation of symptoms is pain in the ear, hearing loss and ringing or buzzing sounds in the ear. Discharge from the ear can be present.

After examination of the ear, the doctor would advise you treatment.

Otitis externa

- Treatment with antibiotic eardrops for 7-10 days. The drops are placed in the ear while the person is lying on his or her side, with the affected ear up.

- In certain cases oral antibiotics may be advised as well.
- Pain medication is given as required
- Protect the ear from water.
- Either an earplug or small cotton ball coated with Vaseline can be used during bathing.

Otitis media

- An oral antibiotic is advised.
- A decongestant medication to be administered.
- Pain medication is given for the first few days.

Toothache

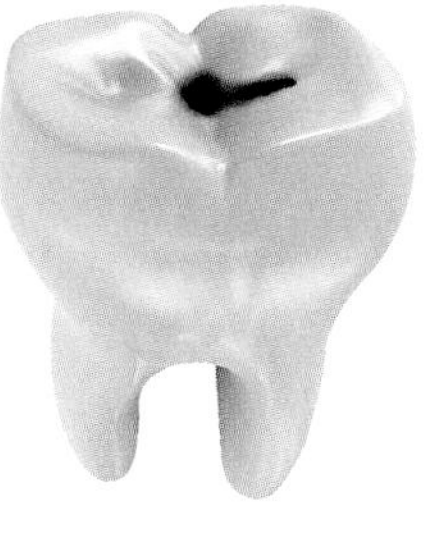

When the nerve root of a tooth is irritated it results in a toothache. Infection, dental abscess, injury, decay, or loss of a tooth are the most common causes of toothache. Tooth pain also occurs after the extraction of a tooth. Other pains which radiate to the jaw and result in tooth pain are ear pain, heart problems or pain in the jaw joint. Molars or wisdom teeth surfacing can also lead to toothache.

Symptoms of toothache

- Hot or cold sensitivity.
- Pain on chewing food.
- Swelling around a tooth or swelling of your jaw.

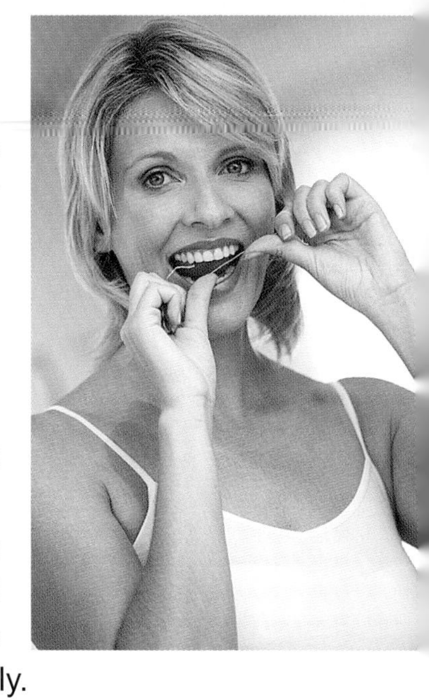

- Bleeding or discharge from around a tooth or gums.
- Injury to the tooth area.

To prevent tooth trouble

- Maintain a healthy diet.
- End your meal with a fibrous fruit.
- It is important to clean your teeth using dental floss every day. Massage and brush your gums daily.
- Prevent tooth decay with fluoride.
- Brush your teeth after every meal.
- Visit your dentist twice a year for check up.

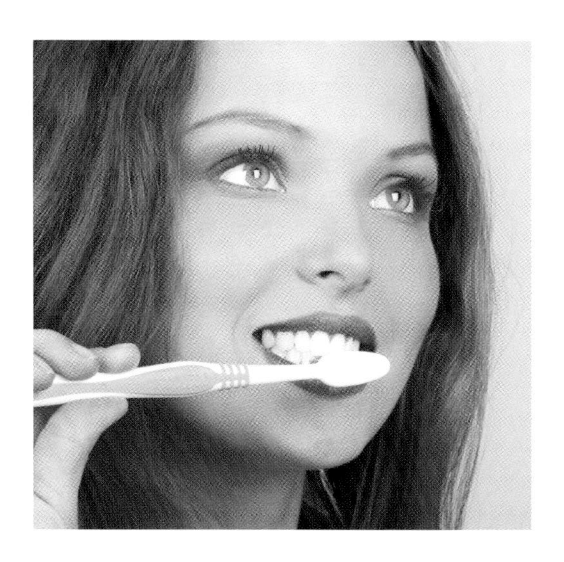

Headache

A headache is a work limiting malady. Majority of headaches are benign and self-limiting. Common causes of a headache can be tension, migraine, eye strain, dehydration, low blood sugar, and sinusitis. The more serious ones can be due to meningitis, encephalitis, cerebral aneurysms, high blood pressure, and brain tumors.Headaches among women can be present during their menstrual years.

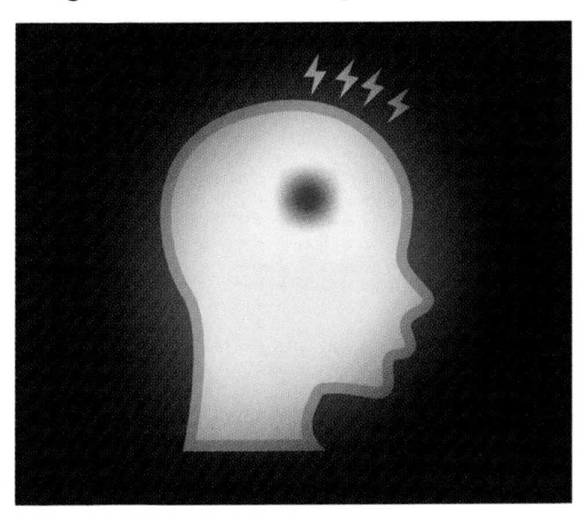

Types of Headaches

- Vascular
- Cervicogenic
- Myogenic (muscle tension)
- Inflammatory

Vascular Headache

A vascular headache is most often called *migraine*. It is characterised by a throbbing or pulsating head and is

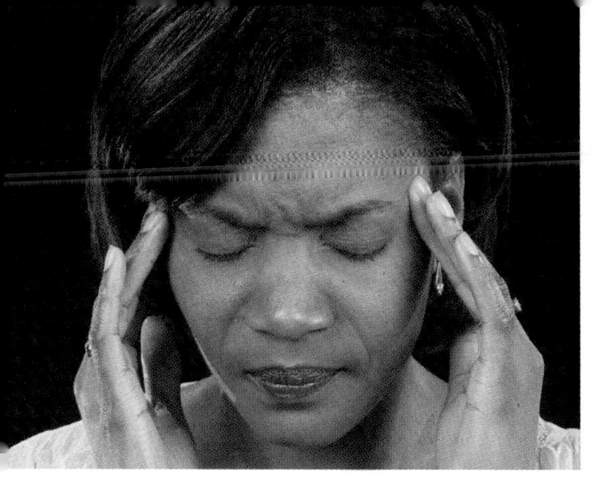

often one sided. It is associated with nausea and vomiting. Sensitivity to light, sound and smells is acute. A vascular headache can lead to depression. There can be a family history of migraine.

Migraine

Triggers off to any stimulus that results in a headache. Stimuli can be:

- Stress
- Environmental factors (e.g. weather, altitude, time zone changes)
- Foods containing caffeine and monosodium glutamate
- Hormonal changes in women
- Lack of sleep
- Alcohol (e.g. red wine)

Some Other Types of Migraine

- **Abdominal migraine** – Most common in children with a family history of migraine. Abdominal pain without a gastrointestinal cause. Nausea, vomiting, and flushing or paleness is seen. Children having abdominal migraine often develop typical migraine as they age.

- **Opthalmoplegic Migraine**
- **Statue Migraine**
- **Carotidynia** or **facial migraine** – It produces deep, dull, aching and sometimes piercing pain in the jaw or neck.
- **Basilar artery migraine** – It involves a disturbance of the basilar artery in the brainstem.

Tension headache

It is the most common form of myogenic headache. Muscular (or myogenic) headaches appear to involve the tightening of muscles. They can radiate to the forehead.

Cervicogenic Headache originates from disorders of the neck (cervical roots C1-C3). This headache is often precipitated by neck movement and/or sustained awkward head positioning.

Inflammatory headache

1. Sinus infection
2. Tension headache
3. Vascular headache
4. Hangover (caused by heavy alcohol consumption)
5. Toxic headache

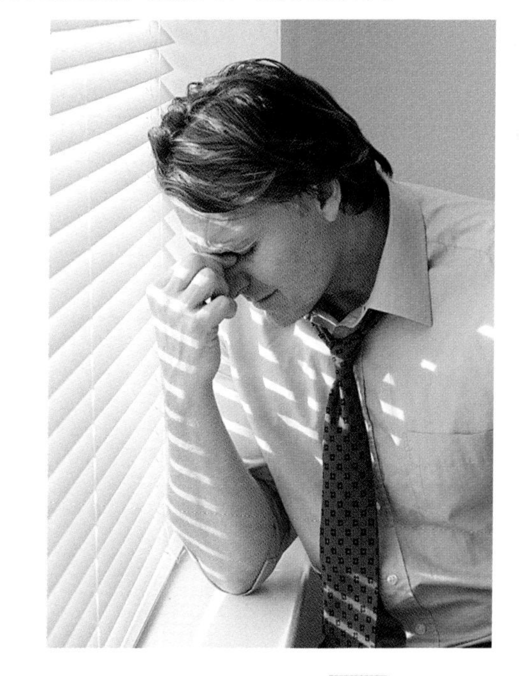

6. Migraine
7. Stroke

Medication

Analgesics provide symptomatic relief from pain. These are usually well-tolerated medication. They are available in oral and injectable forms.

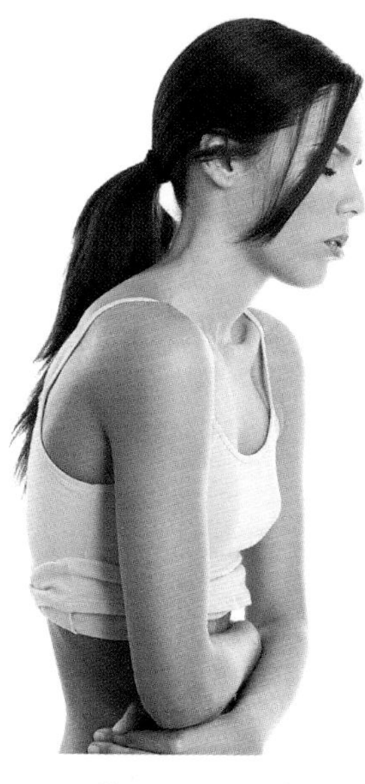

Abdominal Pain in Adults

Abdominal pain is a common problem. Normally this pain is self-limited or cured by home remedies. In serious causes it may require urgent intervention and hospitalisation. Abdominal pain is normally described as acute or chronic. Its nature is defined as sharp, dull or colicky. The area from where the pain arises, its distribution, radiation and other factors are observed to help make a provisional diagnosis.

Causes of Abdominal Pain

- Perforation, e.g. peptic ulcer, diverticulum
- It can be as a result of inflammation (e.g. appendicitis, cholecystitis, pancreatitis)
- Trauma from blunt or perforating injuries of stomach, bowel, spleen etc.

- Obstruction of small bowel and large bowel (due to previous surgery, e.g. colorectal cancer, hernia, etc)

Treatment

- Blood tests including full blood count, electrolytes, urea, creatinine, liver function tests, pregnancy test (in young women) and lipase.
- Urinalysis
- Imaging including erect chest X-ray and plain films of the abdomen.
- An electrocardiograph to rule out a heart attack which can occasionally present as abdominal pain.

If diagnosis of abdominal pain remains unclear after history, examination and basic investigations, then more advanced investigations like computed tomography of the abdomen/pelvis, abdominal or pelvic ultrasound, endoscopy and colonoscopy (not used for diagnosing acute pain) should be included to clinch the diagnosis.

Recurrent abdominal pain in children and adolescents is often due to irritable bowel syndrome

Raynaud's Phenomenon

Raynaud's phenomenon is named after the French doctor Maurice Raynaud. She first described the condition in the mid-1800s. Raynaud's phenomenon results from poor circulation affecting the extremities (i.e., fingers and toes).

In this phenomenon, when an individual's skin is exposed to the cold, the blood vessels under the skin undergo vasospasm (slowing the flow of blood). It then becomes harder for the blood to reach these areas and therefore less oxygen reaches the skin. The skin turns blue and feels cold. The nose and ears may also be affected. Pain in the fingers or toes is experienced when they are cold. A tingling feeling or pain in the fingers or toes when they warm up. Women develop Raynaud's phenomenon more often than men.

Medicines that relax the walls of the blood vessels may be prescribed by your doctor.

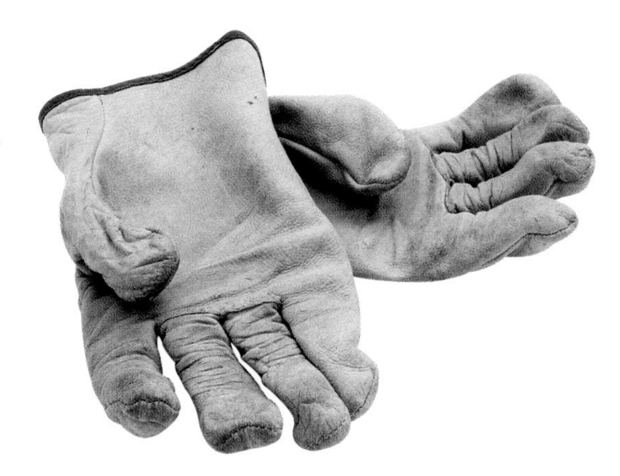

Other Advice

- Keep your hands and feet warm.
- Wear gloves and warm socks in cold weather.
- Do not smoke. Smoking causes blood vessels to constrict, making the symptoms of Raynaud's phenomenon worse. Smoking can also trigger vasospasm in the whole body.

Deep Vein Thrombosis (DVT)

Veins are blood vessels carrying blood towards the heart. When you have a DVT the blood flow in the vein is partially or completely blocked by a thrombus. There can be severe pain in the calf region due to the formation of a thrombus. Blood flow is normally smooth and quick through the veins and does not lead to clotting. Blood flow in the leg veins is helped along by leg movements as muscle action squeezes the veins of the leg. A deep vein thrombosis (DVT) is a result of a blood clot lodging in a deep vein of the leg.

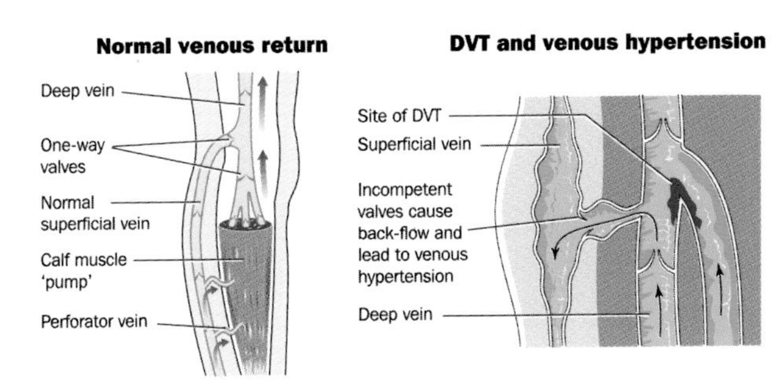

Causes of DVT

- Surgery more than 30 minutes in an individual is the most common cause of DVT. When the patient is under anesthesia, free flow of blood in the leg veins flows down due to no leg movement.
- Any illness or injury that causes immobility increases the risk of DVT.
- Long journeys by plane may cause an increased risk of DVT (especially if the passenger does not move his legs while sitting).

- Vasculitis (inflammation of the vein wall) and some drugs (e.g. chemotherapy drugs) can damage the vein and increase the risk of having a DVT.
- Some medical conditions can cause the blood to clot more readily than usual.

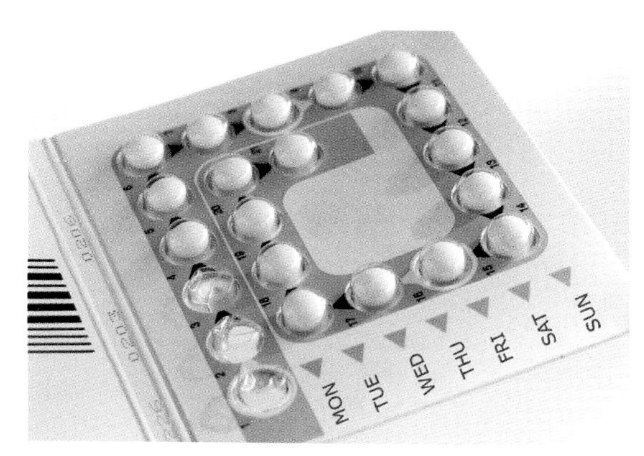

- Hormone replacement therapy (HRT) that contains estrogen can cause the blood to clot. Women taking 'the pill' or 'HRT' are at a greater risk of developing DVT.

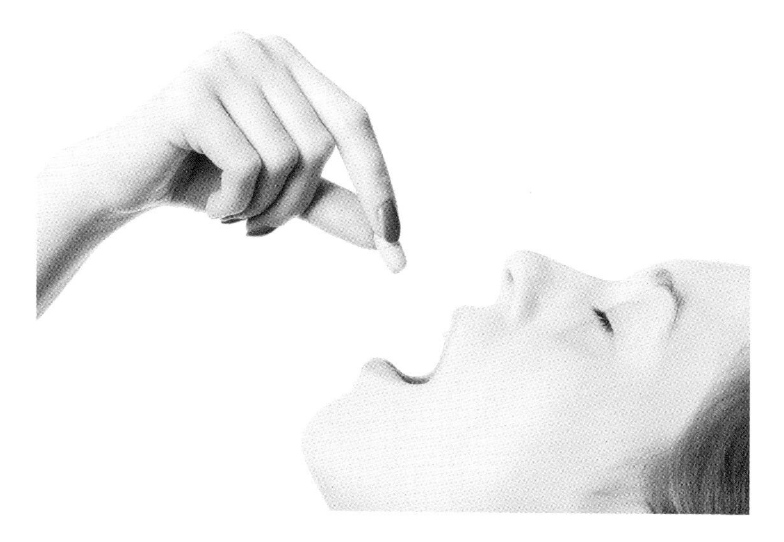

- People with cancer or heart failure have an increased risk of DVT.
- Due to poor mobility, older people are more susceptible to develop DVT.
- Obesity also increases the risk of having an attack of DVT.

Complications of Deep Vein Thrombosis

- Pulmonary embolus (a blood clot that travels to the lung)
- Post-thrombotic syndrome (persistent calf symptoms)

Treatment of Deep Vein Thrombosis

- Anticoagulation to help prevent the clot from getting bigger.
- Compression and raising the leg
- Stop smoking
- Certain tests for clotting time, lipid profile, blood sugar, etc will be advised by your doctor.
- Appropriate medication will then be advised to you.

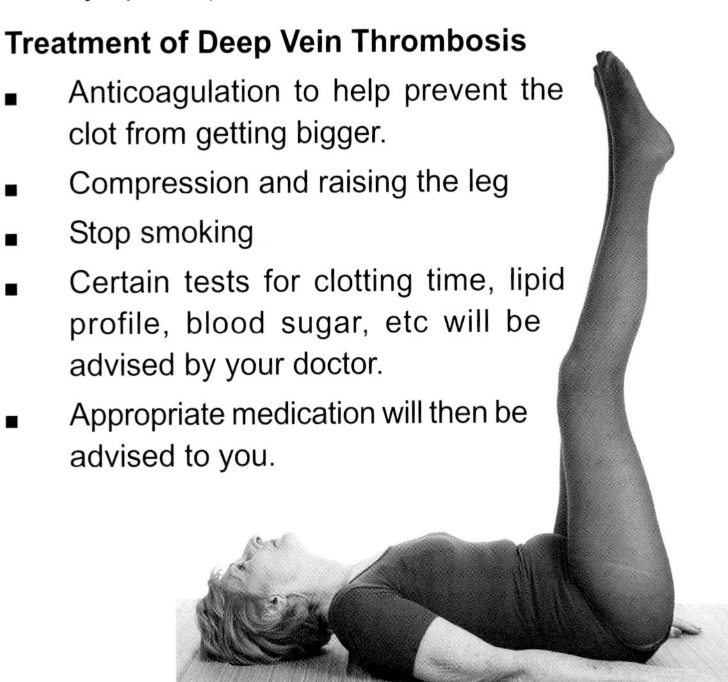

Herpes Zoster

It is commonly known as 'shingles'. It is caused by the *varicella zoster* virus. Chicken pox a short lived illness also occurs due to this virus. Once the episode of chicken pox has resolved, the virus may not get eliminated from the body as it lies in the bodies of the nerve cells. Herpes zoster may occur independently, (without a recent attack of chicken pox).

Symptoms of Herpes Zoster

- Headache, fever and malaise
- These symptoms are often followed by itching and a burning pain.
- Hyperesthesia or parasthesia (i.e. sensitivity to touch, heat, cold etc).

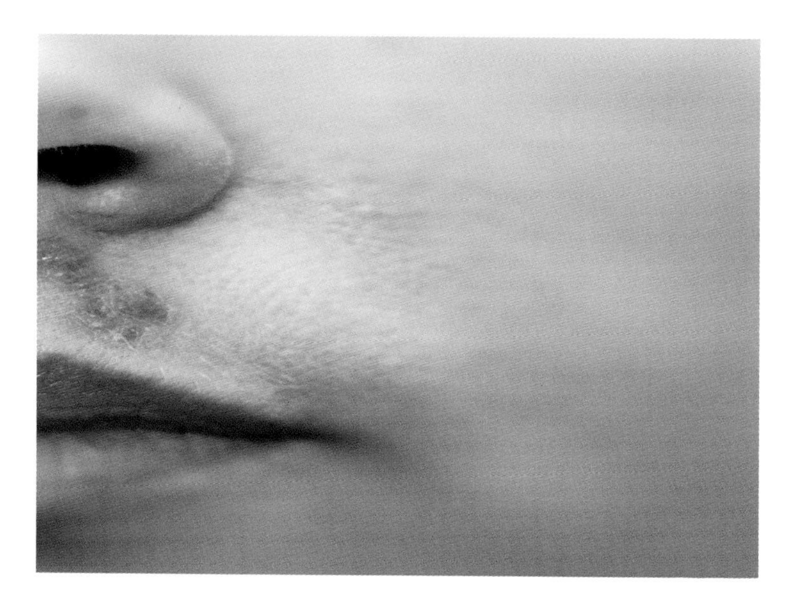

The pain in Herpes Zoster mostly extends along the torso of the body. It can present itself as stinging, tingling and or aching pain. A day or two after the above symptoms, rash appears which can spread to face, eyes, and other parts of the body.

Initially the rash appears in hives, but later it becomes vesicular (in form of small blisters, filled with serous exudate). Fever and general malaise often continue. The painful vesicles become dark as they get filled with blood. About 10 days later, the crust falls off and the skin starts

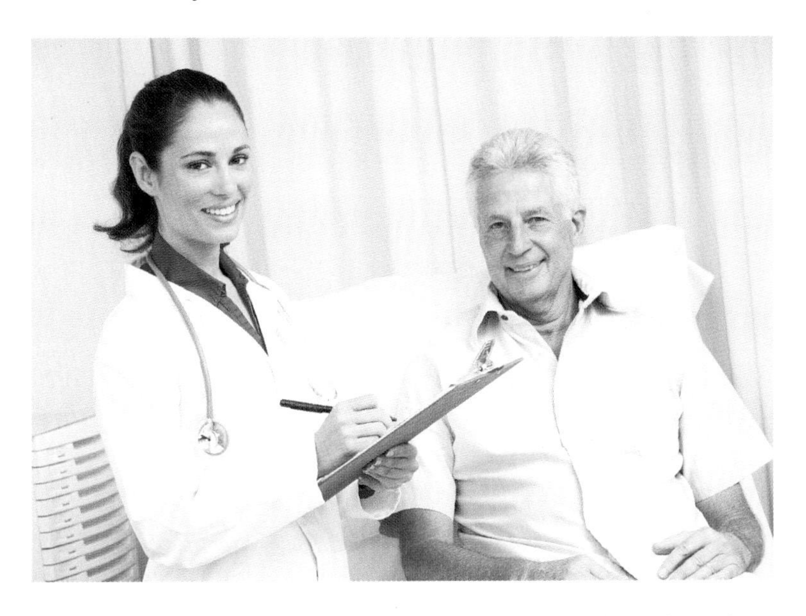

to heal. In case of blistering and scarring discoloration of the skin occurs.

Diagnosis of Herpes Zoster

Laboratory test of this ailment is through a blood sample.

Treatment

- Anti-viral treatment is recommended.
- Oral corticosteroids if required are added to the drug regimen.
- For mild pain analgesics are advised.
- In severe cases opoid medication like morphine can be administered.
- On crusting of lesions, capsaicin cream can be used.

Prevention

Live vaccine for V2V (Zostavar) is used in adults to prevent the disease. Also a study has showed that fresh fruit intake (about three serving a day) helps reduce the risk of developing Herpes Zoster.

Chest pain

Chest pain can be a symptom present due to a number of serious conditions. It could be cardiac in nature and therefore considered a medical emergency. When the chest pain is not associated with heart disease, it is termed as non-cardiac chest pain.

Causes of chest pain

Cardiopulmonary can be

- Angina Pectoris
- Acute coronary syndrome
- Myocardial infarction ("heart attack")
- Aortic dissection

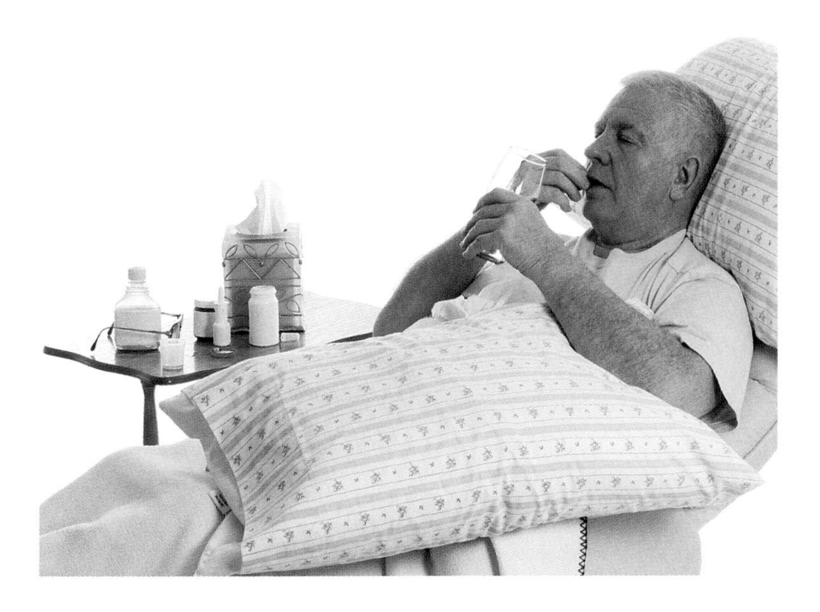

- Pulmonary embolism
- Pneumonia
- Haemothorax

Other causes of chest pain

Upper gastrointestinal diseases e.g. gastroesophageal reflux disease (GERD), Hiatus hernia (which may not accompany GERD) and achalasia cardia.

Others types of chest pain

- Fibromyalgia
- Chest wall problems and breast conditions
- Herpes zoster
- Spinal, nerve problem
- Tietze's syndrome - a benign and harmless form of osteochondritis or costochondritis (often mistaken for heart disease)
- Abdominal pain can also mimic chest pain.

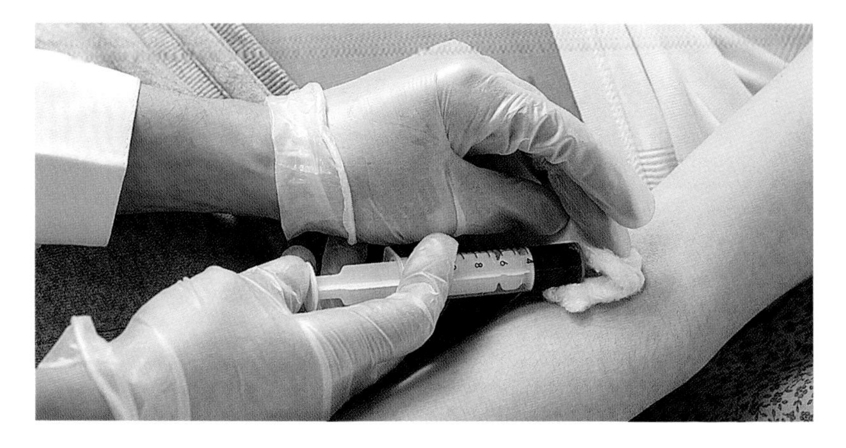

Depending upon the type of pain, a number of tests can be ordered by your doctor

- X-rays of the chest and / or abdomen
- CT Scan
- ECG
- Pulmonary angiogram
- Angiography

Blood tests

- Complete blood count with erythrocyte sedimentation rate (ESR)
- Kidney function test
- Liver function test
- Creatinine kinase

Some other specific tests can also be conducted.

Myths and Fact File

Myth

With arthritis, I do not need to move, just sit

Fact

Along with your medication, a certain amount of mobilization of joints is very important. The more you are immobile, the worse will be your arthritis.

Myth

For osteoporosis the calcium and other medication advised is enough

Fact

To go for a walk is necessary. Mobilization of calcium comes through mobility. Only supplementation of calcium is not enough for proper calcium deposition.

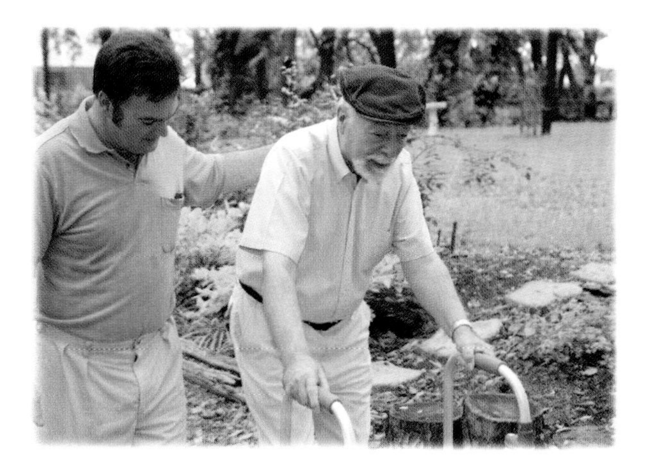

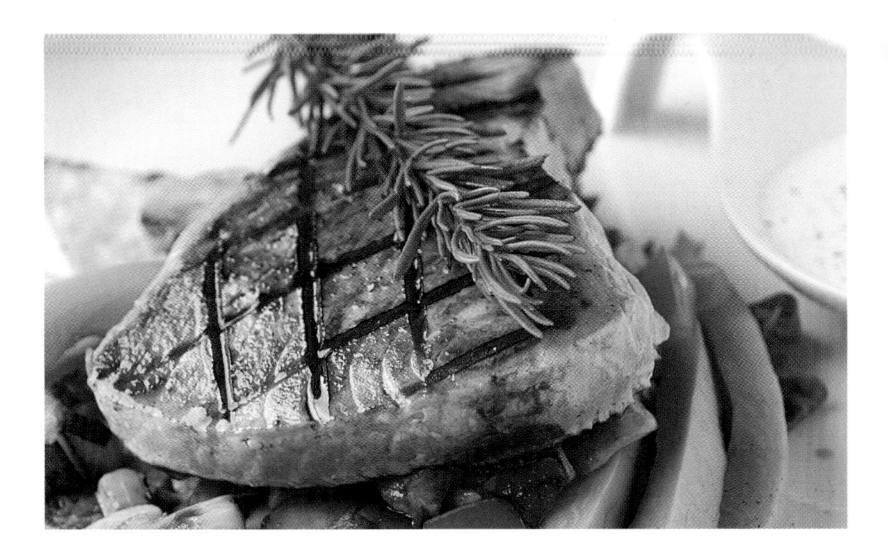

Myth

Osteoporosis is only present in women.

Fact

Osteoporosis can develop in men also. It can occur in anyone with chronic disease, due to certain medication or hormonal disorder.

Myth

Gout runs in families. It has nothing to do with food or drink.

Fact

Gout may or may not be familial. It occurs due to deficiency of an enzyme HGPRtase. Alcohol and high uric acid foods, precipitate the onset of this disease.